INTERMITTENT FASTING 101

THE GUIDE TO INTERMITTENT FASTING HELPS YOU LOSE WEIGHT AND GET LEAN MUSCLE MASS.

Table of contents

Contents

WHAT IS INTERMITTENT FASTING DIET 7

    o   How Does Intermittent Fasting Work? 11

    o   The Benefits of Intermittent Fasting 11

    o   The symptoms of intermittent fasting 14

PROBLEMS OF POOR MODERN DIET **16**

    o   Obesity 18

    o   Hypertension 18

    o   Decreased Production of Blood Cells 18

    o   Elevated Cholesterol and Heart Disease 19

    o   Diabetes 19

    o   Stroke 19

    o   Different impacts are: 20

HOW CAN I FAST ? **22**

    o   Muscle Loss 23

    o   Protein Sparing 24

    o   How to begin intermittent fasting 24

    o   Intermittent fasting is a prevalent method that individuals use to: 25

    o   1. Recognize individual objectives 25

    o   2. Pick the method 25

    o   Eat Stop Eat 26

    o   Warrior Diet 26

    o   Leangains 26

    o   How viable is intermittent fasting 28

    o   Steps to Start Intermittent Fasting 28

    o   Before you begin 29

    o   Address your stresses 30

    o   Tips to help you as the night progressed: 31

    o   Tips to assist you with abstaining from nibbling: 32

    o   6 Popular Ways to Do Intermittent Fasting 34

WHY SHOULD I TRY INTERMITTENT FASTING **38**

    o   How to Start Intermittent Fasting 38

- ○ Types of Intermittent Fasting 39
- ○ The 16:8 Method 39
- ○ The 5:2 Fasting Method 39
- ○ The Eat-Stop-Eat Diet 39
- ○ Substitute Day Fasting.. 39
- ○ The Warrior Diet 39
- ○ The Best Way to Start Intermittent Fasting.. 40

FRUITFUL PARTS OF AN INTERMITTENT FASTING INCLUDE; 42
- ○ Fasting the Best Way to Lose Weight... 42

THE BASIC OF EATING ON AN INTERMITTENT FASTING 44
- ○ For what reason is it advantageous to change when you're eating? 44
- ○ A portion of the indicated health benefits of intermittent fasting include:..... 46
- ○ How Intermittent Fasting Works 47
- ○ The Benefits of Intermittent Fasting 47
- ○ Tips for keeping up intermittent fasting 51

COMMON FITNESS AND NUTRITION MYTHS 54
- ○ The 5 Biggest Myths Surrounding Intermittent Fasting 54

PSYCHOLOGICAL BENEFITS 57

USEFUL RECIPES FOR INTERMITTENT FASTING 60
- ○ Intermittent Fasting Refresher 60
- ○ 12:12 Method 60
- ○ 20:4 Method 60
- ○ 16:8 Method 60
- ○ 5:2 Method 60
- ○ Low-Calorie recipes for the Intermittent Fasting Plan 63

RED CABBAGE AND GREEN APPLE SESAME SLAW.. 72

SMOKY AVOCADO AND JICAMA SALAD 74

MANGO, KALE, AND AVOCADO SALAD 75

STEWED BUTTERNUT SQUASH AND APPLE SOUP 77

CURRIED YELLOW LENTILS WITH AVOCADO "Bread trims." 78

KALE SALAD, APPLES, RAISINS, WITH CARROTS, AND CREAMY CURRY DRESSING 79

RED QUINOA, ALMOND AND ARUGULA SALAD WITH CANTALOUPE 81

HOT THAI SALAD 82

CARROT AVOCADO BISQUE 83

GLUTEN-FREE TORTILLA PIZZA 84

CASHEW CHEESE 85

COOKED CAULIFLOWER AND PARSNIP SOUP 86

HEMP HUMMUS 87

SWEET POTATO HUMMUS 89

TURMERIC TAHINI DRESSING 89

Walnut PESTO 90

Unrefined RANCH DRESSING 91

SMOOTH APRICOT GINGER DRESSING 92

Dim BEAN AND QUINOA SALAD WITH QUICK CUMIN DRESSING 93

ZUCCHINI PASTA WITH, BASIL, SWEET POTATO, HEMP PARMESAN, AND CHERRY TOMATOES 95

o   GLUTEN-FREE WHITE BEAN AND SUMMER VEGETABLE PASTA 96

o   BUTTERNUT SQUASH CURRY 97

o   EGGPLANT ROLLATINI WITH CASHEW CHEESE 100

o   GINGER LIME CHICKPEA SWEET POTATO BURGERS 102

o   SWEET POTATO AND BLACK BEAN CHILI 103

o   CAULIFLOWER RICE WITH LEMON, MINT, AND PISTACHIOS 104

o   DULL COLOURED RICE AND LENTIL SALAD 105

o   ARUGULA SALAD WITH GOJI BERRIES, ROASTED BUTTERNUT SQUASH, AND CAULIFLOWER 107

o   COOKED VEGETABLE PESTO PASTA SALAD 108

o   PORTOBELLO "STEAK" AND CAULIFLOWER "Pureed potatoes." 109

PASTERIES 111

o   BANANA SOFT SERVE 111

o   Rough VEGAN BROWNIE BITES 112

o   Unrefined, VEGAN VANILLA MACAROONS 112

o   CHOCOMOLE 113

o   BLUEBERRY GINGER ICE CREAM 113

THE VEGAN MEAL RECIPES IDEAS 114

o   Kinds of Breakfast plans 114

CONCLUSION 120

Mo **30**	
Di **31**	
Mi **1**	
Do **2**	
Fr **3**	
Sa **4**	
So **5**	

WHAT IS INTERMITTENT FASTING DIET

Intermittent fasting can be defined as a meal plan where you cycle between periods of eating and fasting. It doesn't utter a word about which foods to eat, but instead when you ought to eat them. Intermittent fasting isn't a diet, yet rather a dieting pattern.

In less complex terms: it's creation a cognizant choice to skip certain suppers intentionally.

By fasting and afterward devouring purposely, intermittent fasting for the most part implies that you expend your calories during a particular stretch of the day, and decide not to eat food for a bigger window of time.

Fasting contrasts from starvation in one essential way: control. Starvation is the involuntaryabsence of food for quite a while, prompting extreme affliction or even demise. It is neither purposeful nor controlled.

Fasting, then again, is the intentional retention of food for profound, health, or different reasons. It's finished by somebody who isn't underweight and in this way has enough put away muscle versus fat to live off. Intermittent fasting done right ought not cause enduring, and unquestionably never demise.

Food is effectively accessible, yet you decide not to eat it. It can be for any span of time, from a couple of hours up to a couple of days or – with medicinal supervision – even possibly more than seven days. You may start a fast whenever based on your personal preference, and you may end a fast voluntarily, as well. You can begin or stop a fast in any way, shape or form or no explanation by any means.

Fasting has no standard term, as it is simply the absence of eating.

Whenever that you are not eating, you are intermittently fasting.

Consider the expression "break fast". This alludes to the feast that breaks your fast – which is done day by day.

Intermittent fasting isn't something strange and inquisitive, yet a piece of ordinary, typical life. It is maybe the most seasoned and most dominant dietary mediation possible.

Fasting is the most proficient and predictable system to diminish insulin levels. This was first noted decades back, and generally acknowledged as evident. It is very basic and self-evident. All foods raise insulin, so the best method of lessening insulin is to stay away from all foods. Blood glucose levels stay typical, as the body starts to switch over to consuming fat for vitality. This impact is seen with fasting periods as short as 24-36 hours. Longer span fasts diminish insulin significantly more drastically.

More recently,alternate day by day fasting has been contemplated as a worthy system of diminishing insulin. Customary fasting, notwithstanding lowering insulin levels, has additionally been shown to improve insulin sensitivitysignificantly.This is the missing connection in the weight misfortune astound. Most diets lessen exceptionally insulin-discharging foods, however don't address the insulin opposition issue. Weight is at first lost, however insulin obstruction keeps insulin levels and Body Set Weight high. Fasting is a productive method of diminishing insulin opposition. Lowering insulin frees the group of abundance salt and water. Insulin causes salt and water maintenance in the kidney. Atkins style diets frequently cause diuresis, the loss of abundance water, prompting the conflict that a great part of the underlying weight misfortune is water. While genuine, diuresis is helpful in diminishing swelling, and feeling 'lighter'. Some may likewise take note of a marginally lower pulse. Fasting has likewise been noted to have an early period of quick weight misfortune.

Intermittent fasting revolves around a pattern of eating and fasting periods, that is, times when you don't eat. "Intermittent fasting is the point at which you allow yourself to eat just during a predetermined window of time every day, Glucose and fat are the body's principle wellsprings of vitality. On the off chance that glucose isn't accessible, at that point the body will change by utilizing fat, with no inconvenient health impacts. This is basically a characteristic piece of life. Periods of low food accessibility have consistently been a piece of mankind's history. Systems have developed to adjust to this reality of Paleolithic life. The progress from the fed state to the fasted state happens in a few stages.

1. Feeding – During suppers, insulin levels are raised. This allows take-up of glucose into tissues, for example, the muscle or cerebrum to be utilized legitimately for vitality. Overabundance glucose is put away as glycogen in the liver.

2. The post-absorptive stage – 6-24 hours subsequent to starting fasting. Insulin levels begin to fall. Breakdown of glycogen discharges glucose for vitality. Glycogen stores keep going for around 24 hours.

3. Gluconeogenesis – A 24 hours to a 2 days – The liver makes new glucose from amino acids in a procedure called "gluconeogenesis". Truly, this is interpreted as "making new glucose". In non-diabetic people, glucose levels fall yet remain inside the ordinary range.

4. Ketosis – 2-3 days in the wake of starting fasting – The low degrees of insulin came to during fasting invigorate lipolysis, the breakdown of fat for vitality. The type of fat, known as triglycerides, is broken into the glycerol spine and three unsaturated fat chains. Glycerol is utilized for gluconeogenesis. Unsaturated fats might be utilized for straightforwardly for vitality by numerous tissues in the body, yet not the cerebrum. Ketone bodies, fit for intersection the blood-cerebrum hindrance, are created from unsaturated fats for use by the mind. Following four days of fasting, around 75% of the vitality utilized by the cerebrum is given by ketones. The two significant kinds of ketones created are beta hydroxybutyrate and acetoacetate, which can increment more than 70 crease during fasting.5.Protein protection stage – >5 days – High degrees of development hormone keep up bulk and lean tissues. The vitality for upkeep of basal digestion is primarily met by the utilization of free unsaturated fats and ketones. Expanded norepinephrine (adrenalin) levels avoid the lessening in metabolic rate.The human body has all around created components for managing periods of low food accessibility. Generally, what we are portraying here is the way toward changing from copying glucose (present moment) to copying fat (long haul). Fat is

essentially the body's put away food vitality. In the midst of low food accessibility, put away food is normally discharged to fill the void. So no, the body doesn't 'consume muscle' with an end goal to nourish itself until all the fat stores are utilized.

There are a few distinctive intermittent fasting methods, all of which split the day or week into eating periods and fasting periods.

A great many people effectively "fast" each day, while they rest. Intermittent fasting can be as straightforward as broadening that fast somewhat more.

You can undergo this process by skipping breakfast, eating your first feast around early afternoon and your last supper at 8 pm.

At that point you're actually fasting for 16 hours consistently, and confining your eating to a 8-hour eating window. This is the most famous type of intermittent fasting, known as the 16/8 method.

Regardless of what you may think, intermittent fasting is very simple to do. Numerous individuals report feeling much improved and having more vitality during a fast.

Appetite is generally not excessively enormous of an issue, despite the fact that it tends to be an issue at the outset, while your body is becoming accustomed to not eating for broadened periods.

No food should be eaten during the fasting period, however you can drink water, espresso, tea and other non-caloric refreshments.

A few types of intermittent fasting allow limited quantities of low-calorie foods during the fasting period.

Taking enhancements is for the most part allowed while fasting, as long as there are no calories in them.

Intermittent fasting isn't a diet, it's a pattern of eating. It's a method for booking your dinners with the goal that you benefit from them.

For what reason is it advantageous to change when you're eating?

All things considered, most prominently, it's an incredible method to get lean without going on an insane diet or chopping your calories down to nothing. (A great many people eat greater dinners during a shorter time span.). Intermittent fasting is a strategic method to keep bulk on while getting lean.

With all that stated, the primary explanation individuals attempt intermittent fasting is to lose fat. We'll discuss how intermittent fasting prompts fat misfortune in a minute.

Maybe in particular, intermittent fasting is perhaps the most straightforward methodology we have for dropping terrible weight while keeping great weight on in light of the fact that it requires almost no conduct change.

How Does Intermittent Fasting Work?

To see how intermittent Fasting prompts fat misfortune, we first need to comprehend the contrast between the fed state and the fasted state.

Your body system is in the fed state when it is processing and interesting food. Ordinarily, the eating state begins when you start eating and goes on for three to five hours as your body processes and digests the food you just ate. At the point when you are in the fed express, it's challenging for your body to consume fat because your insulin levels are high.

After that period, your body goes into what is known as the post-absorptive state, which is only an extravagant method for saying that your body isn't preparing a feast. The post-absorptive state goes on until 8 to 12 hours after your last feast, which is the point at which you start the fasted state. It is a lot simpler for your body to consume fat in the fasted state because your insulin levels are low.

At the point when you're in the fasted express, your body can consume fat that has been blocked off during the fed state.

Since we don't start the fasted state until 12 hours after our last supper, fasting places your body system in a fat consuming state, making it to during an ordinary eating plan.

The Benefits of Intermittent Fasting

Fat misfortune is extraordinary. However, it isn't the main advantage of Fasting.

1. Intermittent Fasting fills your heart with joyless complex.

I'm enthusiastic about conduct change, effortlessness, and decreasing pressure. Intermittent Fasting gives extra straightforwardness to my life that I truly appreciate.

2. Intermittent Fasting causes you to live more.

Researchers have since a long time ago realized that limiting calories is a method for extending life. From a legitimate point of view, this bodes well. At the point when you're starving, your body discovers approaches to broaden your life.

Fortunately, intermittent Fasting actuates a large number of indistinguishable instruments for expanding life from calorie limitation. As such, you get the benefits of a more extended existence without the problem of starving.

3. Intermittent Fasting may decrease the risk of malignant growth.

This one is begging to be proven wrong because there hasn't been a ton of experimentation done on the connection between malignant growth and Fasting. Early reports, however, look positive.

4. Intermittent Fasting is a lot simpler than dieting.

The explanation most diets bomb isn't because we change to inappropriate food, this is because we don't follow the diet over the long haul. It is anything but a nutrition issue; it's a conduct change issue.

This is the place intermittent Fasting sparkles since it's surprisingly simple to actualize once you overcome the possibility that you have to eat consistently. Intermittent Fasting was a powerful system for weight misfortune in large grown-ups and reasoned that "subjects rapidly adjust" to an intermittent fasting schedule.

"Diets are simple in the thought, troublesome in the execution. Intermittent Fasting is the polar opposite — it's troublesome in the consideration yet simple in the execution.

A large portion of us has thought about starting to eat less. At the point when we discover a diet that interests us, it appears as though it will be a breeze to do. However, when we get into the quick and dirty of it, it gets intense. So a diet is simple in consideration, however not all that simple in the long haul execution.

Intermittent Fasting is difficult in the examination, of that there is no uncertainty. "You abandon food for 24 hours?" individuals would ask, suspiciously when we clarified what we were doing. "I would never do that." But once begun, it's a simple task. It's extraordinary freedom. Your food uses dive.

What's more, you're not especially ravenous. … Although it's difficult to defeat abandoning food, when you start the routine, nothing could be simpler

On the off chance that is particularly well known in the keto network since it encourages you to consume put away glycogen stores rapidly. That implies getting into ketosis faster.

What's more, getting into ketosis faster is extraordinary news in case you're in the keto-adjustment stage and encountering keto influenza side effects.

The greatest advantage of intermittent Fasting is getting the physiological benefits of calorie limitation without really starving yourself.

At the point when you get into a score with IF, you'll normally eat fewer calories, experience fewer yearnings, and get every one of the benefits of Fasting.

4. You'll adhere to one calendar.

If you've at any point attempted to diet, you likely skill it feels when you tumble off the wagon. While a few people can get right back on, others end up way off-kilter. "In case you're not immaculate and enjoy on dessert, you may think 'alright, I messed up; presently, I will return home and eat that sack of ginger snaps my children left in the bureau. Intermittent Fasting keeps you from going down that hare gap since you're failing to worry about what no doubt about it to eat. Rather, you simply focus on adhering to your fast calendar.

5. You'll enjoy your suppers better.

Regardless of whether you're a rapid eater who indulges before your mind gets the message that you're full or you just never appear to be fulfilled, IF might help. "At the point when you're not eating constantly, your appetite hormones don't should be discharged that regularly," says Jubilee. "The body shows signs of improvement hormonal parity, which empowers you to get a grip on your craving."

6. You'll kick desires for sugary, greasy foods.

Uplifting news in case you're somebody who needs to stop their late-evening eating propensities. Intermittent Fasting can assist you with kicking this unhealthy propensity since it constrains you to quit eating at a specific time. Intermittent Fasting is especially useful for individuals who like to eat foods high in refined carbs and sugar. "Individuals who will, in general, do a great deal of after-supper eating will profit a ton in such a case that encourages them to have more command over this conduct. Also, Intermittent Fasting advances satiety through the creation of more craving lessening hormones. "Following a day or two of Intermittent Fasting, these satiety hormones kick in and will make you feel all the more normally full," she says.

7. You get a back to front hostile to maturing help.

No, it is anything but a fix just for creaky joints, wrinkled skin, or weak hair, however Intermittent Fasting prompts an expansion in human development hormone (HGH), which advances cell fix, not eating for a few backs to back hours makes a slight weight on your cells' mitochondria (the vitality powerhouses), which gives them a bump to fire up their working.

8. If you have pre-diabetes, IF might help get it leveled out.

If your PCP has disclosed to you that you're in peril of creating diabetes, inquire as to whether intermittent Fasting merits an attempt. This sort of eating plan may enable your cells to turn out to be progressively delicate to insulin, says Foroutan. The explanation: Every time you eat, your body discharges the hormone insulin, trying to transport sugar from your circulatory system into your cells for vitality. Individuals who are prediabetic are insulin safe, which means the cells in your body don't react to insulin and it can't take up glucose, so your glucose levels remain raised. Going longer between eating may help since it requires your body to siphon out insulin less regularly.

9. You may bust through a weight misfortune level.

At the point when your weight misfortune endeavors have leveled, IF may serve to kick-start your digestion, says Jubilee. "Your body discovers that if there's no glucose accessible for fuel, there are fat stores to copy for fuel rather," she says.

10. You'll diminish your risk of disease.

Studies show that Intermittent Fasting can help lower your risk of malignancy. That is on the grounds that fasting causes apoptosis, otherwise known as customized cell passing. This implies your body can have progressively steady cell turnover, which averts the potential for disease cells to create, intermittent fasting may have potential anticancer impacts for individuals who are overweight or hefty. Chemotherapy endure treatment better and improve their personal satisfaction. What's more, since you'll have progressively steady cell fix.

Different benefits of Intermittent Fasting include:

• Losing fat while keeping up slender bulk

• Increased human development hormone, which assists with fat misfortune, muscle upkeep and keeping your skin looking youthful

• Improved glucose and insulin levels

• Longevity and insurance from incessant disease

• Increased mind health

The symptoms of intermittent fasting

Much the same as some other weight misfortune diet, intermittent fasting accompanies some reactions. Some of them are sure, such as shedding pounds and getting desires leveled out, while others can be terrible.

1. You may feel aggravated and tired.

At the point when you're skirting a supper, your glucose drops, which can influence your state of mind and vitality levels. Glucose is the primary vitality hotspot for the cerebrum, and when you're not devouring enough calories, your mien can rapidly turn sour. "Individuals may get cerebral pains and feel aggravated so that restricts them from needing to work out or be social.

In any case, one thing you can do to help anticipate this drop in vitality levels is to eat more protein- and fiber-rich dinners with some healthy fats during suppers. That implies stacking up on lean protein, for example, barbecued chicken, salmon, grass-encouraged hamburger, and eggs, in your dishes. There are many plant-based protein alternatives, including quinoa, edamame, and chickpeas, that fill both your protein and fiber needs. Including some healthy fats, for example, avocado and nuts, to your feast can likewise assist you with feeling progressively satisfied.

"Plan your next feast to the point where you know your precise bits, and streamline it with the goal that you're eating foods that will satisfy you.

2. You may feel woozy or tipsy.

Since you're going drawn out hours without food, Intermittent Fasting can cause wooziness and dazedness, which may likewise be indications of hypoglycemia, a condition set apart by low glucose. Some other regular indications of hypoglycemia incorporate weakness, insecurity, perspiring, and a sporadic heartbeat. In case you're inclined to hypoglycemia and are following IF, you ought to be mindful so as to screen your manifestations and work under the supervision of a specialist or enlisted dietitian to avoid enormous dunks in glucose.

Individuals who use insulin, glipizide, or different diabetes medications ought to likewise be administered by their physician if they're following IF. Skipping breakfast or dodging bites can be particularly terrible for individuals with diabetes on the grounds that having predictable dinners avoids spikes in glucose and reinforces the viability of their prescription.

3. Who shouldn't attempt intermittent fasting for weight misfortune?

There are a few people who ought to stay away from intermittent fasting out and out in light of the fact that they live with certain health conditions, take meds that could make Intermittent Fasting hazardous, or have battled with dietary problems previously.

4. You have a dietary problem or have had one before.

Anybody with anorexia or bulimia ought not attempt intermittent fasting. "Individuals with a background marked by dietary problems including confinement or gorging then vomiting ought to stay away from along these lines of eating. "Mentally, it could emulate a limit and gorge stage" and become a trigger for your issue to erupt.

5. If you planned to become pregnant soon.

Ideally this one is an easy decision, however pregnancy isn't normally an opportunity to concentrate on shedding fat, says Jubilee. Except if your primary care physician has trained you generally, center on getting great nutrition for the duration of the day, consistently.

6. You're on medications that should be taken with food in the first part of the day and before bed.

This isn't constantly a major issue, since you may have the option to take a couple of tablespoons of margarine or coconut oil effortlessly their retention without upsetting your stomach or your fasting plan. Talk with your PCP, since Intermittent Fasting may in any case not be the best decision for you.

- ## PROBLEMS OF POOR MODERN DIET

Poor nutrition propensities can be a social health issue, since nutrition and diet influence how you feel, look, think and act. A terrible diet brings about lower center quality, slower critical thinking capacity and muscle reaction time, and less readiness. Poor nutrition makes numerous other negative health impacts too.

The correct foods in the perfect sums are critical to a long and healthy life, and your body's needs change as you get more established. For instance, you don't require the same number of calories, however you need a greater amount of certain nutrients like nutrient D and calcium. What's more, as you age, your body may experience difficulty taking in and utilizing nutrients found in foods, as B12.

Dieteticians has a long history that stretches back at any rate to Hippocrates, who viewed it as for all intents and purposes indivisible from medication. Four of the 10 driving reasons for death in the World today are diet-related conditions – diabetes, coronary illness, stroke and malignancy. The push to drive health care expenses down has urged numerous doctors to move their concentration from the treatment of sicknesses to their counteractive action, which, obviously, includes nutrition. There is no doubt that better nutrition can bring about postponing the beginning of numerous ceaseless maladies and altogether improve the personal satisfaction.

Almost everybody knows about the old nutritional saying that states: "The type of food you eat will affect you general health." This idiom urges you to consider the roots of your food. On the off chance that your food was brought up in a domain loaded with pesticides, herbicides, hereditarily changed living beings (GMOs) and development hormones, it will assimilate those synthetics – thus will you.

Numerous pesticides, for example, DDT, DDE and PCP, have been shown to emulate the impacts of estrogen in the body and have been connected to the developing scourge of estrogen-related health conditions, for example, PMS, bosom malignancy, and low sperm checks.

The EPA, in a proceeding with assessment of pesticides, has so far discovered sixty-four that are conceivably cancer-causing. Numerous others presently can't seem to be tried. Development hormones, for example, rBGH that are found in customarily raised dairy and meat items have been shown to effectsly affect the human body. What's more, the EPA and FDA can not ensure there will be no negative impacts from GMOs. In this day and age, nobody of us can escape contamination totally, however there is a major contrast between the sum and kind of poisons present in natural foods and in those raised by ordinary methods. By picking natural foods, you can altogether diminish the measure of ecological poisons in your body and the earth all in all.

Poor dietary patterns incorporate under-or over-eating, not having enough of the healthy foods we need every day, or expending an excessive number of sorts of food and drink, which are low in fiber or high in fat, salt or potentially sugar.

These unhealthy dietary patterns can influence our nutrient admission, including vitality (or kilojoules) protein, starches, basic unsaturated fats, nutrients and minerals just as fiber and liquid.

Poor nutrition can weaken our day by day health and prosperity and decrease our capacity to lead an agreeable and dynamic life.

Nutrition is the amount and nature of food that the body gets. The body separates the food to get the particles that it very: proteins, fats, sugars, nutrients, and minerals. Nutrition alludes to entirety of all procedures engaged with how creatures acquire nutrients, use them, and use them to help the entirety of life's procedures. On the off chance that body doesn't have these things, than the body will unfit to work appropriately. What's more, the assets of awful nutrition can be horrendous.

Nutrition has been one of the fundamental needs of each individual living on the earth. Nutrition is that procedure which gives vitality to the body to perform different errands in routine life. Various types of sickness, shortcoming and incapacities are closely related with the admission of lacking add up to food nutrients.

Along these lines, more established grown-ups don't generally get the nutrients they need. It may be a smart thought to know the indications of poor nutrition so you can chat with your primary care physician on the off chance that you see any of them.

For the time being, poor nutrition can add to pressure, tiredness and our ability to work, and after some time, it can add to the risk of building up certain sicknesses and other health issues, for example,

Obesity

Obesity is characterized as having a weight file (BMI) of at least 25. Being overweight puts individuals at risk for building up a large group of clutters and conditions, some of them perilous. Being overweight doesn't really mean you're large, and the other way around. Obesitymeans that you have a lot of bodyfat. In case you're overweight you just gauge a lot for your stature, yet the weight can emerge out of muscle and bone. Obesity builds your risk for coronary illness, stroke, diabetes, joint inflammation and some type of malignant growths

There are a few maladies that can cause obesity, yet most of individuals are either idle or settle on poor nutritional decisions and expend an excessive number of calories

Hypertension

Hypertension is one of the potential results of poor nutrition. Hypertension, otherwise called hypertension, is known as the quiet executioner, since it as often as possible stays undetected and in this way untreated until harm to the body has been finished. Eating an excessive amount of shoddy nourishment, singed food, salt, sugar, dairy items, caffeine and refined food can cause hypertension.

Decreased Production of Blood Cells

Pallor happens when you need more red platelets to convey oxygen all through your body. Manifestations of iron deficiency incorporate weakness, affectability to cold temperatures, migraine and a fast, unpredictable heartbeat. Sickliness has different causes, and some are identified with insufficiencies in specific nutrients.

Elevated Cholesterol and Heart Disease

Poor nutrition can prompt elevated cholesterol, which is an essential supporter of coronary illness. Elevated cholesterol foods contain a lot of soaked fat. Models incorporate frozen yogurt, eggs, cheddar, margarine and hamburger. Rather than high fat foods, pick lean proteins, for example, chicken, turkey, fish and seafood and stay away from prepared foods.

Diabetes

Diabetes likewise can be connected to poor nutrition. A few types of the malady can come about because of expending a sugar-and fat-loaded diet, prompting weight gain. As indicated by the National Institute of Health, around 8 percent of the American populace has diabetes.

Improvement of Osteomalacia or Rickets

Osteomalacia and rickets are brought about by an inadequacy of nutrient D, calcium or phosphate. Osteomalacia happens in grown-ups, while rickets happens in kids. Osteomalacia and rickets cause delicate, powerless bones, torment and muscle shortcoming.

Some of the time these sicknesses result from a failure to retain nutrient D or not getting enough daylight so your body can make its very own nutrient D. Nutrient D likewise controls blood levels of calcium and phosphate. These ailments can likewise happen from not getting enough nutrient D, calcium or phosphorus in the diet. These nutrients are found in dairy items, strengthened foods and vegetables. Supplanting the missing nutrients in the diet will alleviate most indications of these maladies.

Stroke

A stroke that is brought about by plaque that develops in a vein, at that point breaks free as a coagulation that movements to your cerebrum and makes a blockage can be connected to poor nutrition. Strokes harm the cerebrum and impede working, once in a while prompting passing. Foods high in salt, fat and cholesterol increment your risk for stroke.

Gout

Poor nutrition can prompt gout. With gout, uric corrosive development brings about the arrangement of gems in your joints. The agonizing expanding related with gout can prompt changeless joint harm. A diet that is high in fat or cholesterol can cause gout. Some seafood- - sardines, mussels, shellfish and scallops- - just as red meat, poultry, pork, spread, entire milk, frozen yogurt and cheddar can expand the measure of uric corrosive in your body, causing gout.

Disease

A few sorts of malignant growth, including bladder, colon and bosom tumors, might be mostly brought about by poor dietary propensities. Farthest point your admission of foods that contains refined sugars, nitrates and hydrogenated oils, including wieners, prepared meats, bacon, doughnuts and french fries.

Different impacts are:

1. Feeling Tired

If you need vitality constantly, it tends to be an indication that you don't get enough of specific nutrients, similar to press. Excessively little of that mineral can prompt iron deficiency - when you need more red platelets to siphon oxygen and nutrients to parts of your body.

Weakness likewise can be an indication of some health conditions, similar to coronary illness or a thyroid issue.

2. Weak, Dry Hair

Nutrients like iron, folate, and nutrient C are significant for your hair. If you don't get enough of these through your diet, you may see some unhealthy changes in it. Your skin likewise may be dainty and pale.

Be that as it may, other health conditions, similar to an issue with your thyroid, can influence your hair and skin, as well.

3. Furrowed or Spoon-Shaped Nails

Poor nutrition can cause a few changes in your nails. Like your hair, your nails can get meager and fragile, yet there can be different signs also. One is nails that bend like a spoon, particularly on your pointer or third finger. That can mean you're low on iron.

Your nails likewise might be furrowed or begin to break into pieces from the nail bed. Notwithstanding issues with iron, nail issues can be brought about by low degrees of protein, calcium, or nutrients A, B6, C, and D.

4. Dental Problems

Your mouth is one of the main spots indications of poor nutrition can show up. An absence of nutrient C can cause the dying, disturbed gums of gum disease (gum infection). If you have dentures or absent or free teeth, that can change your food decisions. Poor nutrition at that point turns into a twofold edged sword: If your mouth damages and you have issues with your teeth, it's much harder to eat healthy foods. Also, that makes it harder to keep your teeth healthy.

5. Change in Bowel Habits

Constipation can occur on the off chance that you don't get enough fiber, found in entire grains, natural products, and vegetables.

6. Mind-set and Mental Health Issues

An unhealthy diet can assume a job in misery. It can influence various mental undertakings and cause you to lose enthusiasm for things you used to appreciate. You additionally may feel bewildered and have memory misfortune.

7. Simple Bruising and Slow Healing

On the off chance that you wound effectively, particularly if there isn't a conspicuous purpose behind it (like falling or finding something), your diet may be having an influence. In particular, you might be inadequate in protein, nutrient C, or nutrient K, which are all expected to mend wounds. Nutrient C encourages tissue to fix itself, and nutrient K is significant for blood coagulating.

8. Slow Immune Response

Without the correct nutrition, your safe framework probably won't be as solid as it should be to battle disease. Probably the most significant nutrients for a solid safe framework are protein and zinc, alongside nutrients A, C, and E.

How to Stay Healthy

The most ideal approach to counteract these sorts of issues is with a decent diet of natural products, vegetables, lean proteins, entire grains, low-fat dairy, and healthier oils. Pick an assortment of these foods at every feast to get the nutrients and minerals you need. Furthermore, attempt to restrain bundled or handled foods and heated merchandise that are high in immersed and trans fats.

• HOW CAN I FAST ?

Fasting is the way toward doing without food for a while to either detox the body or lose weight. Most fasts incorporate drinking water, yet some incorporate abandoning water for a while. During the time spent fasting, the body goes to muscle eventually to get required glucose, which results in loss of bulk. How fast this happens relies upon how a lot of glucose your body is getting. Fasts can be inconvenient to your health, so converse with your primary care physician before beginning one.

People have really been fasting for a large number of years.

Now and again it was done out of need, when there essentially wasn't any food accessible.

In different examples, it was accomplished for strict reasons. Different religions, including Islam, Christianity and Buddhism, order some type of fasting.

People and different creatures likewise regularly instinctually fast when wiped out.

Unmistakably, there is not all that much about fasting, and our bodies are very well prepared to deal with broadened periods of not eating.

A wide range of procedures in the body change when we don't eat for some time, so as to allow our bodies to flourish during a period of starvation. It has to do with hormones, qualities and significant cell fix forms.

When fasted, we get huge decreases in glucose and insulin levels, just as an exceptional increment in human development hormone.

Numerous individuals do intermittent fasting so as to lose weight, as it is an exceptionally straightforward and compelling approach to confine calories and consume fat.

Metabolic health benefits, as it can improve different diverse risk variables and health markers.

There is additionally some proof that intermittent fasting can assist you with living longer. Concentrates in rodents show that it can expand life expectancy as successfully as calorie confinement.

Some examination likewise proposes that it can help ensure against ailments, including coronary illness, type 2 diabetes, malignancy, Alzheimer's ailment and others.

Other individuals essentially like the accommodation of intermittent fasting.

It is a compelling "life hack" that makes your life more straightforward, while improving your health simultaneously. The less suppers you have to plan for, the less complex your life will be.

Not eating 3-4+ times each day (with the readiness and cleaning included) additionally spares time.

If you are on a water-just fast, a few key changes will occur. The body needs certain essential parts, typically gave by diet, to work, the most significant of which is glucose. When the body takes everything it can from the last dinner you had, it goes to the liver, which stores glucose as glycogen. It takes around 24 hours before the liver is soothed of its glycogen stores.

Muscle Loss

When the glycogen stores of the liver run out after the initial 24 hours, the body goes to unsaturated fats for fuel, separating the unsaturated fats in the stores of fat in the body and around the organs. In any case, different pieces of the body, fundamentally the mind and red platelets, can just capacity utilizing glucose. The body takes the glucose from glycerol in the fat tissues and the amino acids in muscle, accordingly starting the procedure of muscle weakening.

Protein Sparing

Sooner or later, more often than not between 48 to 72 hours after the beginning of the fast, the body understands that taking glucose from the muscles is excessively inefficient. The body at that point experiences a procedure known as ketosis, where the liver produces ketone bodies from unsaturated fats that the mind can use as fuel; just the red platelets will keep utilizing the muscles for fuel. This diminishes the sum the muscles are utilized as fuel essentially and is alluded to as "protein saving." After 72 hours, ketosis proceeds as long as there is sufficient fat in the body. Drawn out fasting can prompt a state set apart by hurtful degrees of ketone bodies and significant levels of sharpness in the blood. Ketosis more often than not begins following 48 hours for ladies and 72 hours for men. Note that ketosis is not quite the same as ketoacidosis. Ketosis is normally a controlled state, set about by low-starch consumption. Ketoacidosis discharges unquestionably more ketone bodies and is regularly a consequence of uncontrolled diabetes.

The vast majority begin to lose bulk following 24 to 48 hours. To stop the procedure, or if nothing else lessen it, devouring a fluid with glucose, more often than not as sugar can help. Squeezes and sports drinks with glucose are a prominent decision. Protein shakes can likewise help. A type of fluid fasting for large patients so as to kick off their weight misfortune. Counsel with a specialist before starting a fasting routine.

How to begin intermittent fasting

Believe you're prepared to try intermittent fasting out? Make sure to counsel your physician or an enrolled dietitian to assist you with finding the best IF plan that accommodates your health and nutrition needs—and to guarantee that it won't influence any prescriptions you're taking or intensify any current health issues.

Numerous individuals who need to attempt IF pick the 16:8 method since it allows you to eat anything you desire for an eight-hour window and afterward fasting for 16 hours. In the fasting period, you can drink water, tea, espresso, and even diet pop. Try to make sense of what eight-hour eating window works best for you. Is it proper to say that you are fine with skipping breakfast? Or do you work out in the first part of the day and want to swear off supper? Examination with the eating and fasting interims that work best for you. However, similar to every prohibitive diet, there are a few downsides. For one, drinking charged beverages while fasting can upset your circadian cadence, and in this way, your digestion.

On the off chance that may not additionally be a long haul answer for keeping up weight misfortune, as it very well may be trying to have a public activity and appreciate eating out and social occasions, which aren't helpful for a period limited method for eating. On the off chance that this diet isn't working for you, converse with your PCP about following kind of eating plan that accommodates your way of life and health needs.

Intermittent fasting includes cycling between periods of eating and fasting. From the outset, individuals may think that its hard to eat during a short window of time every day or shift back and forth between long periods of eating and not eating. This article offers tips on the most ideal approach to start fasting, including distinguishing individual objectives, planning suppers, and setting up caloric needs.

Intermittent fasting is a prevalent method that individuals use to:

- simplify their life

- lose weight

- improve their general health and prosperity, for example, limiting the impacts of maturing

In spite of the fact that fasting is alright for most healthy, well-sustained individuals, it may not be suitable for people who have any ailments. For those prepared to begin fasting, the following tips intend to assist them with making the experience as simple and effective as could be allowed.

1. Recognize individual objectives

Normally, an individual who starts intermittent fasting has an objective as a primary concern. It might be to lose weight, improve by and large health, or improve metabolic health. An individual's definitive objective will assist them with deciding the most appropriate fasting method and work out what number calories and nutrients they have to expend.

2. Pick the method

Regularly, an individual should stay with one fasting method for a month or longer before attempting another.

There are four potential methods that an individual may attempt when fasting for health reasons. An individual should pick the plan that suits their inclinations and which they want to stay with.

These include:

- Eat Stop Eat

- Warrior Diet

- Leangains

- Alternate Day Fasting

Ordinarily, an individual should stay with one fasting method for a month or longer to check whether it works for them before attempting an alternate method. Any individual who has an ailment should converse with their healthcare supplier before starting any fasting method.

When settling on a method, an individual ought to recall that they don't have to eat a specific sum or kind of food or stay away from foods out and out. An individual can eat what they need. However, to arrive at health and weight misfortune objectives, it is a smart thought to follow a high-fiber, vegetable-rich diet during the eating times.

Gorging on unhealthful foods on eating days can thwart health progress. It is likewise critical to drink bunches of water or other no-calorie refreshments all through the fast days.

Eat Stop Eat

Eat Stop Eat is a form of fasting method that includes eating nothing for 24 hours two times every week. It doesn't make a difference what days an individual fasts or in any event, when they start. The main confinement is fasting must keep going for 24 hours and on non-back to back days.

Individuals who don't eat for 24 hours will probably turn out to be exceptionally ravenous. Eat Stop Eat might not be the best method for individuals who are new to fasting to begin with.

Warrior Diet

An individual fasting along these lines expends all their regular food consumption in the staying 4 hours.

Eating an entire day of food in such a brief span can make an individual's stomach very awkward. This is the most outrageous fasting method, and also to Eat Stop Eat, an individual new to fasting might not have any desire to begin with this method.

Leangains

Leangains are for weightlifters, yet it has picked up fame among other individuals who are keen on fasting. Not at all like Eat Stop Eat and the Warrior Diet, fasting for Leangains includes a lot shorter periods.

For instance, guys who pick the Leangains method will fast for 16 hours and afterward eat what they need for the staying 8 hours a day. Females can fast for 14 hours and eat what they need for the staying 10 hours of the day.

During the fast, an individual must abstain from eating any food yet can drink the same number of no-calorie refreshments as they like.

Exchange Day Fasting, 5:2 method

A few people fast on exchange days to improve glucose, cholesterol, and weight misfortune. An individual on the 5:2 method eats 500 to 600 calories on two non-continuous days every week.

Some other day fasting regimens include a third day of fasting every week. For the remainder of the week, an individual eats just the quantity of calories they consume during the day. After some time, this makes a calorie shortage that allows the individual to lose weight.

3. Make sense of caloric needs

There are no dietary limitations when fasting, yet this doesn't mean calories don't check.

Individuals who are hoping to lose weight need to make a calorie shortfall for themselves — this implies they devour less vitality than they use. People that are hoping to put on weight need to devour a bigger number of calories than they use.

There are numerous apparatuses accessible to enable an individual to work out their caloric needs and decide what number calories they have to expend every day to either put on or lose weight. An individual could likewise address their healthcare supplier or dietitian for direction on what number calories they need.

4. Make sense of a supper plan

An individual keen on losing or putting on weight may discover it plans what they will eat during the day or week.

Dinner planning shouldn't be excessively prohibitive. It thinks about calorie consumption and consolidating legitimate nutrients into the diet.

Dinner planning offers numerous benefits, for example, helping an individual adhere to their calorie check, and guaranteeing they have the important food close by for cooking plans, speedy suppers, and bites.

5. Make the most of the calories

Not all calories are the equivalent. Despite the fact that these fasting methods don't set confinements on what number calories an individual ought to devour when fasting, it is fundamental to think about the nutritional estimation of the food.

An individual should mean to eat nutrient-thick food, or food with a high concentration of nutrients per calorie. Despite the fact that an individual might not need to relinquish low quality nourishment completely, they should in any case practice control and spotlight on progressively healthful alternatives to pick up the most benefits.

How viable is intermittent fasting

Fasting effectsly affects an individual's body. These impacts include:

- Reducing levels of insulin, which makes it simpler for the body to utilize put away fat.

- Lowering blood sugars, circulatory strain, and aggravation levels.

- Changing the statement of specific qualities, which enables the body to shield itself from sickness just as advancing life span.

- Dramatically builds human development hormone, or HGH, which enables the body to use muscle versus fat and develop muscle.

- The body actuates a recuperating procedure specialists call autophagy, which basically implies that the body processes or reuses old or harmed cell parts.

Fasting goes back to old people who frequently went hours or days between suppers as acquiring food was troublesome. The human body adjusted to this style of eating, allowing stretched out periods to go between food admission times.

Intermittent fasting reproduces this constrained fasting. At the point when an individual attempts an intermittent fast for dietary proposes, it very well may be viable for weight misfortune. Indeed, a great many people attempt intermittent fasting to help lose weight.

Numerous individuals who fast observe a higher loss of instinctive muscle versus fat and a like marginally less decrease in body weight contrasted and individuals who follow progressively conventional calorie decrease diets.

Steps to Start Intermittent Fasting

- Someone online is ready to end on a positive note on day 2 of her multi day fast since she's not by any means hungry. However, rather than getting persuaded you state "It's just 10

AM and I'm as of now eager as a greedy monster, I won't last the entire day, I can't do this today."

- Hunger aches and longings were so solid you didn't make it. "It's simpler to fast when that is no joke," the specialists state. However, that takes a little while on a low carb diet and you would prefer not to hold up that long.

- Maybe you haven't attempted it, however you've pondered it. "Goodness, I can't do that."

Imagine a situation in which there was a quiet and certain approach to begin. Furthermore, consider the possibility that your present capacities were sufficient.

Here's how:

Instead of considering it to be another troublesome obligation you owe to your health, make it a self-explore.

- Break it down into little yet effectively feasible bit by bit activities that assurance you will wrap up,
- observe and investigate what you find,
- draw your decision: Is fasting directly for you?

So you're not focusing on it, you're here to find out about it. Since like the vast majority, you learn by doing. Doesn't that sound simpler as of now? In any case…

Before you begin

1. Cosult your primary care physician before you start. Particularly in the event that you have any ailment or in case you're on any medicine. Stop in the event that you feel wiped out.

2. Keep it basic. Fasting (in this investigation) is characterized as expending just plain water (level or carbonated), or dark espresso, or unsweetened tea.

3.   Keep it simple. Eat your typical suppers during your eating window. As far as I can tell, intermittent fasting works best when joined with a low carb-high fat diet of genuine, entire foods. However, propelling the ideal blend to get the best outcomes isn't your objective at this moment… it's to complete a fast.

4.   Time (for example 7 PM) is referenced for straightforwardness. You don't need to follow them. You may modify the occasions as indicated by your timetable.

5.   Which days of the week? As far as I can tell, fasting on weekdays are increasingly helpful in light of the fact that they're progressively organized and have less factors. In any case, that may not be valid for you. What you're searching for are those days where you're bound to state, "Where'd the time go? I neglected to eat!"

6.   Slip ups are alright. To begin with, excuse yourself. You may get the latest relevant point of interest or start from Day 1.

For what reason would you like to attempt intermittent fasting? How might this benefit you?

•   Weight misfortune, weight upkeep. Fasting diminishes hormones, for example, insulin, and builds HGH and norepinephrine which causes put away muscle to fat ratio increasingly open to consume for vitality, so you lose fat.

•   Avoid drug, mitigate side effects. Fasting causes you forestall diabetes, coronary illness, decrease irritation.

•   Prevent genuine ailment, life span. Studies show fasting may give assurance against Alzheimer's, malignancy, and may assist you with living longer.

Consider the reasons why you settled on this decision when you feel "denied".

Address your stresses

What will make you anxious about intermittent fasting that it makes you stop?

- It's alright to skip breakfast. It's not the most significant feast of the day, it's an unbiased supper, there's nothing valuable about it. Truly, skipping breakfast won't make you put on weight and having breakfast won't start up your digestion.

- It's alright to maintain a strategic distance from snacks. Nibbling won't assist you with getting more fit since it doesn't help your digestion. Truth be told, this examination shows nibbling adds to obesity and greasy liver illness.

- Your digestion won't slow down. Fasting really expands your digestion and encourages you hold more muscle while getting thinner.

There's no motivation to be fearful in light of the fact that it's not dangerous to your health.

Day 1, don't have after supper

Eat your standard suppers for the duration of the day, yet quit having after supper.

It's far-fetched that you're extremely eager around 8-9 PM after you had supper at 7 PM. What's more, it more often than not accompanies popcorn, chips, or frozen yogurt.

Tips to help you as the night progressed:

- Get a glass of water or a warm cup of quieting home grown tea as opposed to eating food.

- Brush your teeth. The minty taste can help check yearnings. It likewise sends a subliminal message that you're finished eating for the afternoon or you'd need to brush your teeth once more. It's a sufficient boundary that can shield you from eating.

Day 2, Delay breakfast

Hello! You simply did a 12-hour fast.

Your last dinner was at 7 PM the previous evening, and it's presently 7 AM. That is 12 hours. You didn't eat for a large portion of a day. You've balancedeating and fasting to a proportion of 50:50, 12 hours of eating and another 12 hours of fasting. This is something worth being thankful for.

That wasn't so difficult, would it say it was? All you needed to do was quit having after supper. Time passes quickly when you're resting!

Delay breakfast today. Eat it when it's helpful. Have water, espresso, or tea.

There's nothing extraordinary about postponing your first supper of the day until it's helpful. Like after you've landed at the workplace or the children have been dropped off to class rather than in the midst of the distraught morning surge.

After you get the chance to work, settle in. Browse your email, take a gander at your schedule, plan your day. You don't need to sneak in breakfast previously or eat while you're doing this.

- 10 AM. It's an ideal opportunity to make the most of your breakfast without the turmoil.

- 12 early afternoon. Noon. You're most likely not eager since you just ate. The clock says it's noon yet your body doesn't say as much. It's alright to hold back to eat until you feel hungry once more.

- 2 PM. You're ravenous currently, have a pleasant lunch.

Have supper at 7 PM.

Develop on the earlier advances: Don't have after supper, defer breakfast until 10 AM.

Day 3, Don't nibble

Very much done! You simply did a 15-hour fast.

You ate at 7 PM the previous evening, quit having after supper, and deferred breakfast until 10 AM. After lunch today, don't have until supper.

Tips to assist you with abstaining from nibbling:

- Dinner's just a couple of hours away. You realize you will eat soon. You should simply pause.

- Hunger comes in waves. It's transitory, it won't deteriorate over the long haul, it will die down.

- The craving may not be genuine. Possibly you're parched. Perhaps it's an early evening time nibbling propensity. Perhaps you're focused, restless, stressed, miserable, or exhausted so you're constrained to eat. Drink water, espresso, or tea.

- Stay occupied. Do some work, a task, go for a stroll, or call a companion. Before you know it, it's a great opportunity to make a beeline for the supper that anticipates you.

Eat at 7 PM.

Develop on the earlier advances: don't have after supper, postpone breakfast until 10 AM, don't nibble in the middle of dinners.

Day 4, Avoid breakfast.

If you did a 15-hour fast – and you didn't nibble…congrats.

You ate at 7 PM the previous evening, quit having after supper, deferred breakfast until 10 AM, and you didn't nibble among lunch and supper.

- You rehearsed careful eating when you didn't eat while doing another action.

- You abstained from eating out of thirst, propensity, or feeling when you held back to eat until you genuinely felt hungry.

- You felt hunger as brief. Do the stunts that helped you ride appetite waves until they left.

Have supper at 7 PM.

Develop on the earlier advances: don't have after supper, skip breakfast, don't nibble in the middle of lunch and supper.

Day 5, Repeat the process

Congrats! You simply did a 16-hour fast.

You ate at 7 PM the previous evening, you skipped breakfast by eating your first feast at 11 AM, didn't nibble, didn't eat again until 7 PM.

It's an intermittent fasting convention called the 16/8 Method advanced by Martin Berkhan. It has a few varieties. It's prominent on the grounds that the vast majority of us aren't really ravenous toward the beginning of the day so it's anything but difficult to skip breakfast.

Your eating window is diminished to ⅓ of the day (8 hours). You've tipped the scale toward a more noteworthy fasting window of ⅔ of the day (16 hours). The helpful impacts kick in.

Progress to other broadened varieties of intermittent fasting. Apply the rule of separating the fast into little however effectively feasible strides over some undefined time frame and stir your way up until you arrive.

6 Popular Ways to Do Intermittent Fasting

Intermittent fasting has been very in vogue as of late.

It is professed to cause weight misfortune, improve metabolic health and maybe even broaden life expectancy.

As anyone might expect given the prevalence, a few unique sorts/methods of intermittent fasting have been concocted.

Every one of them can be successful, however which one fits best will rely upon the person.

Here are 6 famous approaches to practice Intermittent fasting Diets.

1. The 16/8 Method Fasting: Fasting for 16 hours each and every day.

The 16/8 Method includes fasting each day for 14-16 hours, and confining your day by day "eating window" to 8-10 hours.

Inside the eating window, you can fit in 2, 3 or more suppers.

Doing this method of fasting can really be as basic as not having anything after supper, and skipping breakfast.

For instance, if you finish your last dinner at 8 pm and, at that point don't eat until 12 early afternoon the following day, at that point you are in fact fasting for 16 hours between suppers.

It is prescribed that ladies just fast 14-15 hours, since they appear to improve somewhat shorter fasts.

For individuals who get eager toward the beginning of the day and like to have breakfast, at that point this can be difficult to become accustomed to from the start. However, many breakfast captains entirely eat thusly.

You can drink water, espresso and other non-caloric refreshments during the fast, and this can help diminish craving levels.

It is imperative to eat generally healthy foods during your eating window. This won't work on the off chance that you eat loads of low quality nourishment or extreme measures of calories.

2. The 5:2 Diet method; Fast for 2 days out of every week.

The 5:2 diet includes eating regularly 5 days of the week, while confining calories to 500-600 on two days of the week.

On the fasting days, it is suggested that ladies eat 500 calories, and men 600 calories.

For instance, you may eat regularly on all days with the exception of Mondays and Thursdays, where you eat two little suppers (250 calories for every feast for ladies, and 300 for men).

As pundits accurately bring up, there are no investigations testing the 5:2 diet itself, however there are a lot of nutrients on the benefits of intermittent fasting.

3. Eat-Stop-Eat: Do a 24-hour fast, more than once per week.

Eat-Stop-Eat includes a 24-hour fast, either more than once every week.

By fasting from supper one day, to supper the following, this adds up to a 24-hour fast.

For instance, if you finish supper on Monday at 7 pm, and don't have until supper the following day at 7 pm, at that point you've quite recently done an entire 24-hour fast.

You can likewise fast from breakfast to breakfast, or lunch to lunch. The final product is the equivalent.

Water, espresso and other non-caloric refreshments are allowed during the fast, yet no strong food.

If you are doing this to reduce your weight, at that point it is significant that you eat typically during the eating periods. As in, eat a similar measure of food as though you hadn't been fasting by any stretch of the imagination.

The issue with this method is that an entire 24-hour fast can be genuinely hard for some individuals.

However, you don't have to bet everything immediately, beginning with 14-16 hours and afterward moving upwards from that point is fine.

4. Interchange Day Fasting: Fast every other day.

Interchange Day fasting means fasting each other day.

There are a few unique adaptations of this. Some of them allow around 500 calories during the fasting days.

A large number of the lab studies showing health benefits of intermittent fasting utilized some adaptation of this. A full fast every other day appears to be fairly extraordinary, so I don't prescribe this for learners.

With this method, you will hit the hay hungry a few times each week, which isn't extremely charming and most likely unsustainable in the long haul.

5. The Warrior Diet Method; Fasting during the day, eat a gigantic feast around evening time.

It includes eating limited quantities of crude foods grown from the ground during the day, at that point eating one immense supper around evening time.

Fundamentally, you "fast" throughout the day and "blowout" around evening time inside a 4 hour eating window.

The Warrior Diet was one of the primary well known "diets" to incorporate a type of intermittent fasting. This diet likewise accentuates food decisions that are very like a paleo diet - entire, natural foods that take after what they resembled in nature.

6. Unconstrained Meal Skipping: Skip suppers when helpful.

You don't really need to follow an organized intermittent fasting plan to receive a portion of the rewards.

Another alternative is to just skip dinners every once in a while, when you don't feel hungry or are too occupied to even think about cooking and eat.

It is a legend that individuals need to eat like clockwork or they will hit "starvation mode" or lose muscle. The human body is well prepared to deal with significant stretches of starvation, not to mention missing a couple of suppers every now and then.

So in case you're truly not eager one day, skip breakfast and simply have a healthy lunch and supper. Or if in case you're voyaging some place and can't discover anything you need to eat, do a short fast.

Avoiding 1 or 2 dinners when you feel so slanted is essentially an unconstrained intermittent fast.

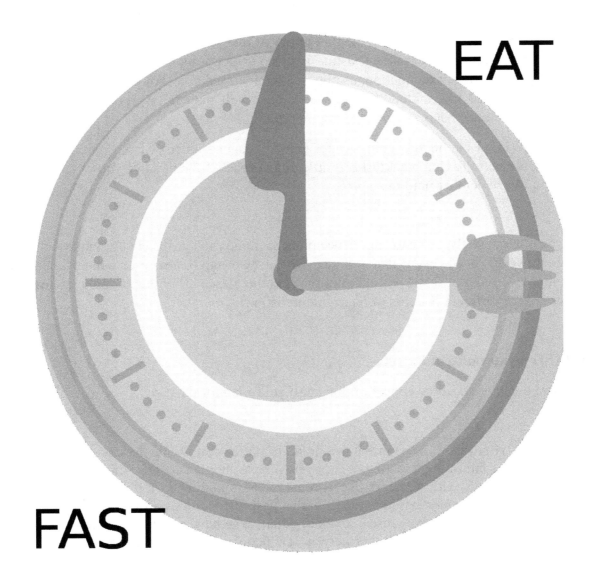

EAT

FAST

• WHY SHOULD I TRY INTERMITTENT FASTING

So you need to begin intermittent fasting. Intermittent fasting is in excess of a dieting craze and has increased genuine prominence as of late because of its significant impacts on weight misfortune and body structure. Fasting has likewise ascended to acclaim in view of its underwriting from the science network, where regarded and fruitful analysts tout its health benefits on the heart, cerebrum and essentially every other organ.

Prior to diving in, it's critical to see precisely what intermittent fasting, implies. In least difficult terms, intermittent fasting is a dietary calendar that includes eating just during explicit timespans and not eating outside of what is normally known as the "bolstering window."

A great many people get hung up on the possibility of intermittent fasting, Since it appears to be excessively troublesome. Intermittent fasting isn't too troublesome in the event that you treat the program as a fun dietary examination, as opposed to an errand you should attempt to get healthy. Nobody needs to do intermittent fasting, yet it very well may be a ground-breaking weight-misfortune apparatus whenever executed appropriately.

Truly, you're (in all likelihood) going to get greedily eager sooner or later, particularly in case you're accustomed to having breakfast and little dinners each 2-3 hours like you were told to do as long as you can remember unto this point.

Truly, you're most likely going to experience plunges, jumps and drops in your vitality, center and stamina. However, in the event that you stay with it, you may likewise encounter improvedfat-consuming, lowered glucose levels andimproved insulin affectability, improvedheart health2 and an entire host of different benefits of intermittent fasting.

How to Start Intermittent Fasting

Before you begin, mark these couple of things off your plan for the day:

- Ask your PCP if intermittent fasting is alright for you. While the vast majority are great to give intermittent fasting, a go, a few people shouldn't. Those gatherings incorporate individuals with ailments like coronary illness and Type 1 diabetes, ladies who are pregnant or lactating, individuals with a past filled with disarranged eating, individuals who are constantly focused, and individuals who have never tried different things with a calorie limitation. Furthermore, a few people who are exceptionally dynamic may locate that intermittent fasting meddles with their athletic performance4.

- Take a second look at your calendar. Does your work/school/life timetable allow you to effortlessly execute intermittent fasting? In the event that you normally meet with partners for supper and breakfast, it may be difficult to set up a predictable sustaining window.

- Mentally set yourself up. In case you're a novice to intermittent fasting, realize that you most likely won't get it immaculate the first (or initial not many) times around. Practice self-pardoning now, before any slip-ups cause you weakening self-blame.

Types of Intermittent Fasting

There are a few conventions for intermittent fasting, each with its own gathering of evangelists.

The 16:8 Method

One of the most famous is the 16:8 method, where followers eat the entirety of their food in a 8-hour window and fast for the staying 16 hours of the day. This is regularly the most straightforward convention for learners to follow in light of the fact that for 7-8 of those 16 fasting hours, you ought to be sleeping.

The 5:2 Fasting Method

Another famous intermittent fasting, convention is the 5:2 diet, which includes eating regularly on five days of the week and confining calorie admission to just 500-600 calories on the other two days. Numerous individuals who follow the 5:2 diet fast on Mondays and Thursdays to separate the week moderately uniformly.

The Eat-Stop-Eat Diet

The appropriately named eat-stop-eat method is an intermittent fasting, convention that includes a total 24-hour fast more than once per week. A typical method to follow eat-stop-eat is to fast starting with one supper then onto the next.

Substitute Day Fasting

Interchange day fasting is an intermittent fasting, method in which followers eat ordinarily one day, fast the following, etc. Fasting for this situation frequently means eating just 500-600 calories on the fasting day, instead of complete caloric confinement.

The Warrior Diet

The Warrior Diet: is another type of intermittent fasting that includes fasting for the duration of the day and truly devouring during a 4-hour window around evening time.

The Best Way to Start Intermittent Fasting

Ok, the brilliant inquiry. Much the same as whatever else in health and wellness, there's nobody most ideal approach to begin intermittent fasting. Truly: You're simply must try it out. Be that as it may, to set yourself up for an effective first fast, follow these means:

1.   Establish your nourishing cutoff. The ideal strategies to do this is to think about what time you ordinarily have supper. On the off chance that you eat your last huge feast at 6 p.m., start your fasting at exactly at 6:30 p.m. You may stare at that announcement in case you're accustomed to relaxing on the lounge chair with popcorn or whatever your night kryptonite is. Be that as it may, inquire as to whether you are extremely ravenous an hour or two after supper, or in case you're simply eating without much forethought.

2.   Consider what time you wake up. In the event that you wake up at 6:30 a.m., well done! You can without much of a stretch total a 12-hour fast.

3.   Think about when you typically have breakfast. Do you will in general surge out the entryway pushing a granola bar in your mouth? Assuming this is the case, ask yourself what the fact of the matter is. Once more, observe whether you're extremely eager or in case you're scooping breakfast since you've been revealed to it's the best activity since preschool. Rather, take a stab at holding up until 10 a.m. or on the other hand so to eat a light tidbit.

From that point, start altering your sustaining window to one that works for you. For the good of simplicity, utilize the 16:8 convention for instance. Eating around 10 a.m. to 6 p.m. may work for you, on the off chance that you work ordinary 9-5 hours. The most ideal approach to begin intermittent fasting is to set up an encouraging window that works with a mind-blowing remainder, not against it.

Analysis with various kinds of intermittent fasting to discover what works best for your way of life. Numerous individuals consider the 16:8 convention the least complex and most reasonable type of intermittent fasting. Start with the 16:8 method and proceed onward to progressively confused conventions as you feel increasingly great with fasting and your body adjusts.

It might take seven days to 10 days to change in accordance with this new eating pattern. From the start, you'll likely feel hungry toward the beginning of the day in light of the fact that the hormone ghrelin, which manages your yearning patterns, causes your body to long for food simultaneously every day.

Would you be able to Drink Water When Intermittent Fasting?

Truly. Truth be told, you're urged to drink more water than expected when intermittent fasting, particularly during the fasting periods. Drinking water stifles yearnings and craving during fasting periods, and is especially useful for amateurs.

Star tip: Drink additional water while fasting to make up for the hydration that you ordinarily get from food. Include a teaspoon of pink Himalayan salt to each liter of water to help relieve flushing and renew mineral levels.

Drinking additional water is likewise basic since you'll likely be eating less food than expected, and up to 20 percent of your every day water admission originates from the food you eat. So in case you're intermittent fasting and haven't increased your water admission, take a couple of drinks before you accuse cerebrum haze or weakness for the fasting convention.

Would you be able to Drink Coffee While Intermittent Fasting?

Another significant yes! Espresso is allowed during both fasting and devouring periods of intermittent fasting conventions. Be that as it may, note that during your fasting periods, you can't include sugar or any type of milk or half and half. Elective zero-calorie sugars like Stevia are alright, yet they may add to yearnings during fasting periods.

While you can drink espresso during intermittent fasting, attempt to abstain from getting subject to it as an approach to fight off yearnings or episodes of exhaustion. Rather, evaluate what and when you ate the day preceding to check whether any changes may help. You can likewise drink unsweetened teas and zero-calorie refreshments like Powerade Zero or Vitamin Water Zero, yet be cautioned that satisfactory flavors may escalate yearnings.

How to Be Successful with Intermittent Fasting

Numerous individuals don't discover accomplishment with intermittent fasting since they utilize their encouraging periods as chances to eat anything they desire. And keeping in mind that you may feel like you've earned some shoddy nourishment in the wake of fasting for 16, 24, or more hours, the impacts of that on your weight-misfortune objectives will outlive the dopamine impact from delectable food.

FRUITFUL PARTS OF AN INTERMITTENT FASTING INCLUDE;

1. Calories: If you're attempting to lose weight, despite everything you have to keep up a caloric shortage. Do whatever it takes not to redress (intentionally or something else) for missed calories during your sustaining windows.

2. Food quality: Just on the grounds that you're confining your eating window, doesn't mean you have free rule with food decisions. Entire, nutrient-thick foods will consistently deliver the best results.

3. Consistency: Intermittent fasting isn't a get-thin snappy plan. Similarly as with any healthy, economical weight-misfortune method, fasting requires devotion.

4. Self-trustworthiness: Don't anticipate that fasting should be simple from the outset. You've presumably spent most of your life eating the right things when you're ravenous or at whatever point you feel like it.

Fasting the Best Way to Lose Weight

The benefits of fasting are dumbfounding. Intermittent fasting decreases insulin opposition, secures against some incessant and degenerative diseases3, can improve heart health and makes healthy eating simpler for certain individuals. In any case, there are blended surveys about its effect on weight misfortune.

However, some examination focuses to hormonal changes produce by fasting that outcome in intense weight misfortune. Fasting reliably and consistently lowers insulin levels and raises both development hormone and norepinephrine levels. As a result of those hormonal changes, fasting can expand your metabolic rate.

Steady fasting likewise enables your body to turn out to be increasingly fat-adjusted, which means you become progressively effective at consuming muscle to fat ratio for fuel, instead of the food you as of late ate. This is frequently called flipping the metabolic switch.

Intermittent fasting can be a useful apparatus for weight misfortune whenever done appropriately. Intermittent fasting can reduce up to 8 percent weight misfortune more than 3-24 weeks. That equivalent investigation additionally found that individuals on INTERMITTENT FASTING, conventions lost 4-7 percent of their midriff boundary, which is one pointer that fasting accompanies more health benefits than weight misfortune. If not done appropriately — for instance, indulging during bolstering periods — INTERMITTENT FASTING won't prompt weight misfortune any superior to another method.

Fasting can likewise make healthy eating simpler, in light of the fact that you have less choices to make and reduce the time to make awful ones. Planning, getting ready and tidying up following 2-3 suppers for every day is a lot simpler than doing the entirety of that for 4-6 dinners.

The greatest admonition about intermittent fasting, however, is that it can meddle with business and social relations in a badly arranged manner. You're bound to be effective with fasting in case you're single, don't have a family, and don't work in a customer confronting business. Since eating is an instilled social movement, you will more than likely face ungainly circumstances wherein you should deny food as a result of your fasting convention.

Much the same as any weight-misfortune method, intermittent fasting works for a few and doesn't work for other people. If you like the possibility of INTERMITTENT FASTING what's more, you don't fall under any class of individuals who shouldn't attempt intermittent fasting, at that point give it a go. If you don't care for the possibility of INTERMITTENT FASTING, at that point you can securely forego the counsel in this article and keep eating such that works for you.

• THE BASIC OF EATING ON AN INTERMITTENT FASTING

Intermittent fasting isn't a diet, it's a pattern of eating. It's a method for booking your suppers with the goal that you benefit from them. Intermittent fasting change not what you eat, it changes when you actually eat them.

For what reason is it advantageous to change when you're eating?

All things considered, most eminently, it's an incredible method to get lean without going on an insane diet or chopping your calories down to nothing. Indeed, more often than not you'll attempt to keep your calories a similar when you start intermittent fasting. (A great many people eat greater suppers during a short period.) Additionally, intermittent fasting is a decent method to keep bulk on while getting lean.

With all that stated, the principle reason individuals attempt intermittent fasting is to lose fat. We'll discuss how intermittent fasting prompts fat misfortune in a minute.

Maybe above all, intermittent fasting is probably the least difficult system we have for dropping awful weight while keeping great weight on in light of the fact that it requires almost no conduct change. This is a generally excellent thing since it implies intermittent fasting falls into the class of "straightforward enough that you'll really do it, however significant enough that it will really have any kind of effect."

Realize this is typical and people have advanced to fast for shorter timeframes – hours or days – without impeding health outcomes. Muscle to fat ratio is just food vitality that has been put away. In the event that you don't eat, your body will basically "eat" its very own fat for vitality.

Life is about parity. The great and the awful, the yin and the yang. The equivalent applies to eating and fasting. Fasting, all things considered, is essentially the other side of eating. If you deprive yourself of eating, you are fasting. Here's how it functions:

At the point when we eat, more food vitality is ingested than can quickly be utilized. A portion of this vitality must be put away for later use. Insulin is the key hormone engaged with the capacity of food vitality.

Insulin rises when we eat, putting away the overabundance vitality in two separate ways. Starches are separated into singular glucose (sugar) units, which can be connected into long ties to shape glycogen, which is then put away in the liver or muscle.

There is, however, exceptionally constrained extra room for starches; and once that is come to, the liver begins to transform the abundance glucose into fat. This procedure is called once more lipogenesis (which means actually "making new fat").

A portion of this recently made fat is put away in the liver, however its vast majority is sent out to other fat stores in the body. While this is an increasingly confounded procedure, there is no restriction to the measure of fat that can be made.

In this way, two corresponding food vitality stockpiling frameworks exist in our bodies. One is effectively open however with constrained extra room (glycogen), and the other is progressively hard to get to yet has practically boundless extra room (muscle to fat ratio).

The procedure goes backward when we don't eat (intermittent fasting). Insulin levels fall, flagging the body to begin consuming put away vitality as no more is coming through food. Blood glucose falls, so the body should now destroy glucose out of capacity to consume for vitality.

Glycogen is the most effectively available vitality source. It is separated into glucose particles to give vitality to the body's different cells. This can give enough vitality to control a great part of the body's requirements for 24-36 hours. From that point onward, the body will essentially be separating fat for vitality.

So the body just truly exists in two states – the fed (insulin high) state and the fasted (insulin low) state. It is possible that we are putting away food vitality (expanding stores), or we are consuming put away vitality (diminishing stores). It's either. In the event that eating and fasting are adjusted, at that point there ought to be no net weight change.

On the off chance that we start eating the moment we turn up, and don't stop until we rest, we invest practically the entirety of our energy in the fed state. After some time, we may put on weight, since we have not allowed our body whenever to consume put away food vitality.

To reestablish harmony or to lose weight, we may basically need to build the measure of time spent consuming food vitality. That is intermittent fasting.

Generally, intermittent fasting allows the body to utilize its put away vitality. The significant thing to comprehend is that there is nothing amiss with that. That is how our bodies are structured. That is the thing that pooches, felines, lions and bears do. That is the thing that people do.

In the event that you are eating each third hour, as is regularly prescribed, at that point your body will continually utilize the approaching food vitality. It will not have to consume a lot of muscle to fat ratio, assuming any. You may simply be putting away fat. Your body might be sparing it for when there is nothing to eat.

If this occurs, you need balance. You need intermittent fasting.

Fasting has no standard term, as it is only the nonattendance of eating. Whenever that you are not eating, you are intermittently fasting. For instance, you may fast among supper and breakfast the following day, a period of around 12-14 hours. In that sense, intermittent fasting ought to be viewed as a piece of regular daily existence.

Consider the expression "breakfast". This alludes to the supper that breaks your fast – which is done every day. As opposed to being a type of remorseless and surprising discipline, the English language certainly recognizes that fasting ought to be performed day by day, regardless of whether just for a brief term.

Intermittent fasting isn't something strange and inquisitive, however a piece of regular, typical life. It is maybe the most established and most dominant dietary mediation possible. However somehow we have missed its capacity and disregarded its restorative potential.

Figuring out how to fast appropriately give us the alternative of utilizing it or not.

Intermittent fasting's most evident advantage is weight misfortune. However, there are a numerous potential benefits past this, some of which have been known since old occasions.

The fasting periods were regularly called 'washes down', 'detoxifications', or 'sanitizations', yet the thought is comparative – for example to keep away from eating food for a specific period of time, regularly for health reasons. Individuals envisioned that this period of forbearance from food would clear their bodies' frameworks of poisons and restore them.

A portion of the indicated health benefits of intermittent fasting include:

- Weight and muscle versus fat misfortune
- Increased fat consuming
- Lowered blood insulin and sugar levels
- Possibly inversion of type 2 diabetes
- Possibly improved mental lucidity and fixation
- Possibly expanded vitality
- Possibly expanded development hormone, at any rate for the time being
- Possibly an improved blood cholesterol profile
- Possibly longer life
- Possibly actuation of cell purging by invigorating autophagy
- Possibly decrease of irritation

Fasting offers numerous significant extraordinary favorable circumstances that are not accessible in commonplace diets.

Where diets can confuse life, intermittent fasting may improve it. Where diets can be costly, intermittent fasting can be free. Where diets can require significant investment, fasting spares time. Where diets might be restricted in their accessibility, fasting is accessible anyplace. What's more, as examined prior, fasting is a conceivably amazing method for lowering insulin and diminishing body weight.

How Intermittent Fasting Works

To see how intermittent fasting prompts fat misfortune we first need to comprehend the distinction between the eating mode and the fasted mode.

Your body system is in the fed state when it is processing and engrossing food. Regularly, the fed state begins when you start eating and goes on for three to five hours as your body processes and assimilates the food you just ate. At the point when you are in the fed express, it's extremely difficult for your body to consume fat if your insulin levels has increased.

The post–absorptive state goes on until 8 to 12 hours after your last supper, which is the point at which you start fasting state. It is a lot simpler for you body to consume fat in the fasting state if your insulin levels are low.

At the point when you're in the fasted express your body can consume fat that has been out of reach during the eatimng mode.

Since we don't enter the fasted mode until 12 hours after our last dinner, it's uncommon that our bodies system are in this fat consuming state. This is a reason why numerous individuals who start intermittent fasting will lose fat without changing what they eat and how much they eat it, or how frequently they work out. Fasting places your body in a fat consuming state that you seldom make it to during a typical eating plan.

The Benefits of Intermittent Fasting

Fat misfortune is extraordinary, yet it isn't the main advantage of fasting.

1. Intermittent fasting fills your heart with joy less difficult.

I'm enthusiastic about conduct change, straightforwardness, and decreasing pressure. Intermittent fasting gives extra effortlessness to my life that I truly appreciate.

2. Intermittent fasting causes you live more.

Researchers have since a long time ago realized that confining calories is a method for stretching life. From a consistent point of view, this bodes well. At the point when you're fasting, your body develops approaches to expand your life.

There's only one point: who needs to starve themselves for the sake of living longer?

I don't mnd you, yet I'm keen on appreciating a long life. Starving myself doesn't sound that inviting.

Fortunately intermittent fasting enacts huge numbers of indistinguishable instruments for broadening life from calorie confinement. As it were, you get the benefits of a more drawn out existence without the issue of starving.

3. Intermittent fasting may decrease the risk of malignant growth.

This one is easy to refute in light of the fact that there hasn't been a great deal of research and experimentation done on the connection among malignancy and fasting. Early reports, however, look positive.

4. Intermittent fasting is a lot simpler than dieting.

The explanation most diets bomb isn't on the grounds that we change to an inappropriate foods, this is because we don't really follow the diet over the long haul. It is anything but a nutrition issue, it's a conduct change issue.

This is the place intermittent fasting sparkles since it's astoundingly simple to execute immediatrely. Intermittent fasting was a powerful system for weight misfortune in hefty grown-ups and inferred that "subjects rapidly adjust" to an intermittent fasting schedule.

There are a wide range of methods for intermittent fasting. The methods fluctuate in the quantity of fast days and the calorie allowances.

There are different approaches to intermittent fasting, and individuals will lean toward various styles. Peruse on to get some answers concerning seven distinct approaches to do intermittent fasting.

1. Fast for 12 hours per day

Various styles of intermittent fasting may suit various individuals. The guidelines for this diet are basic. An individual needs to settle on and cling to a 12-hour fasting window consistently.

As per a few specialists, fasting for 10–16 hours can causeTrusted Source the body to transform its fat stores into vitality, which discharges ketones into the circulatory system. This ought to energize weight misfortune.

This sort of intermittent fasting plan might be a decent choice for novices. This is on the grounds that the fasting window is generally little, a significant part of the fasting happens during rest, and the individual can expend a similar number of calories every day.

The most effortless approach to do the 12-hour fast is to incorporate the period of rest in the fasting window.

For instance, an individual could fast between 7 p.m. furthermore, 7 a.m. They would need to complete their supper before 7 p.m. what's more, hold up until 7 a.m. to have breakfast however would be snoozing for a great part of the time in the middle.

2. Fasting for 16 hours

Having Fasted for 16 hours per day, leaving an eating window of 8 hours, is known as the 16:8 fasting method or the leangains diet.

At the point of 16:8 diet, men fast for 16 hours every day, and ladies fast for 14 hours. This sort of intermittent fast might be useful for somebody who has just attempted the 12-hour fast yet didn't perceive any benefits.

On this fast, individuals more often than not complete their night supper by 8 p.m. and afterward skip breakfast the following day, not eating again until early afternoon.

Restricting the nourishing window to 8 hours shielded them from obesity, aggravation, diabetes, and liver ailment, in any event, when they ate indistinguishable absolute number of calories from mice that ate at whatever point they wished.

3. Fasting for 2 days every week

Individuals following the 5:2 diet eat standard measures of healthful food for 5 days and diminish calorie admission on the other 2 days.

During the 2 fasting days, men for the most part devour 600 calories and ladies 500 calories.

Commonly, individuals separate their fasting days in the week. For instance, they may fast on a Monday and Thursday and eat typically on different days. There should be at any rate 1 non-fasting day between fasting days.

The impacts of this fasting style in 23 overweight ladies. Through the span of one menstrual cycle, the ladies lost 4.8 percent of their body weight and 8.0 percent of their all out muscle to fat ratio. However, these estimations came back to typical for the vast majority of the ladies following 5 days of ordinary eating.

4. Substitute day fasting

There are a few varieties of the other day fasting plan, which includes fasting each other day.

For certain individuals, substitute day fasting implies a total shirking of strong foods on fasting days, while other individuals allow up to 500 calories. On encouraging days, individuals regularly eat as much as they need.

Substitute day fasting is a serious outrageous type of intermittent fasting, and it may not be appropriate for fledglings or those with certain ailments. It might likewise be hard to keep up this sort of fasting in the long haul.

5. A week after week 24-hour fast

On a 24-hour diet, an individual can have teas and sans calorie drinks. Fasting totally for 1 or 2 days per week, known as the Eat-Stop-Eat diet, includes eating no food for 24 hours one after another. Numerous individuals fast from breakfast to breakfast or lunch to lunch.

Individuals on this diet plan can have water, tea, and other without calorie drinks during the fasting period.

Individuals should come back to typical eating patterns on the non-fasting days. Eating as such lessens an individual's absolute calorie admission however doesn't restrain the particular foods that the individual devours.

A 24-hour fast can be testing, and it might cause weakness, cerebral pains, or peevishness. Numerous individuals find that these impacts become less outrageous after some time as the body acclimates to this new pattern of eating.

Individuals may profit by attempting a 12-hour or 16-hour fast before progressing to the 24-hour fast.

6. Feast skipping

This adaptable way to deal with intermittent fasting might be useful for novices. It includes once in a while skipping dinners.

Individuals can choose which suppers to skirt as indicated by their degree of appetite or time limitations. However, it is critical to eat healthful foods at every dinner.

Feast skipping is probably going to be best when people screen and react to their body's craving signals. Basically, individuals utilizing this style of intermittent fasting will eat when they are eager and skip dinners when they are definitely not.

This may feel more normal for certain individuals than the other fasting methods.

7. The Warrior Diet

The Warrior Diet is a moderately outrageous type of intermittent fasting. The Warrior Diet includes eating practically nothing, generally only a couple of servings of crude products of the soil, during a 20-hour fasting window, at that point eating one huge feast around evening time. The eating window is normally just around 4 hours.

This type of fasting might be best for individuals who have attempted different types of intermittent fasting as of now.

Supporters of the Warrior Diet guarantee that people are normal nighttime eaters and that eating around evening time allows the body to pick up nutrients in accordance with its circadian rhythms.

During the 4-hour eating stage, individuals should ensure that they devour a lot of vegetables, proteins, and healthful fats. They ought to likewise incorporate a few starches.

It is conceivable to eat a few foods during the fasting period, it tends to challenge to adhere to the severe rules on when and what to eat in the long haul. Additionally, a few people battle with eating such an enormous feast so close to sleep time.

There is likewise a risk that individuals on this diet won't eat enough nutrients, for example, fiber. This can build the risk of malignant growth and adversy affect stomach related and insusceptible health.

Tips for keeping up intermittent fasting

Yoga and light exercise may make intermittent fasting simpler.

It tends to challenge to adhere to an intermittent fasting program.

The following tips may assist individuals with remaining on track and boost the benefits of intermittent fasting:

- Staying hydrated. Drink bunches of water and sans calorie drinks, for example, natural teas, for the duration of the day.

- Avoiding fixating on food. Plan a lot of interruptions on fasting days to abstain from contemplating food, for example, getting up to speed with desk work or heading out to see a motion picture.

- Resting and unwinding. Maintain a strategic distance from strenuous exercises on fasting days, albeit light exercise, for example, yoga might be useful.

- Making each calorie check. In the event that the picked plan allows a few calories during fasting periods, select nutrient-thick foods that are concentrated in protein, fiber, and healthful fats. Models incorporate beans, lentils, eggs, fish, nuts, and avocado.

- Eating high-volume foods. Select filling yet low-calorie foods, which incorporate popcorn, crude vegetables, and natural products with high water content, for example, grapes and melon.

- Increasing the taste without the calories. Season dinners liberally with garlic, herbs, flavors, or vinegar. These foods are amazingly low in calories yet are loaded with season, which may decrease sentiments of appetite.

- Choosing nutrient-thick foods after the fasting period. Consuming foods that are high in fiber, nutrients, minerals, and different nutrients keeps glucose levels unfaltering and avert nutrient lacks. A decent diet will likewise add to weight misfortune and generally speaking health.ing intermittent fast required.

10. Regard your body signs.

Focus on what your body lets you know.

This incorporates:

- drastic changes in hunger, yearning, and satiety – including food longings;

- sleep quality;
- energy levels and athletic execution;
- mood and mental/passionate health;
- immunity;
- blood profile;
- hormonal health; and,
- how you look.

11. Exercise, however, don't try too hard.

We emphatically prescribe you consolidate practice with IF to take advantage of it. Don't try too hard. See #12.

12. Think of what is going on in your life.

Consider:

- how much exercise/preparing you do, and how seriously;
- how well you rest and recoup;
- how well IF is fitting into your standard daily practice and typical social exercises; and,
- what different requests and stress life offers you.

Keep in mind: IF is one of the numerous nutrition styles that work. Be that as it may, it possibly "works" when it's intermittent, adaptable, and part of your ordinary everyday practice – not a commitment, and not a continuous wellspring of physical and mental pressure

• COMMON FITNESS AND NUTRITION MYTHS

The 5 Biggest Myths Surrounding Intermittent Fasting

Intermittent fasting is one of the most mainstream health and wellness points today. You may have known about it from a companion or watched a cool video on the web. How about we jump further into the study of intermittent fasting to show signs of improvement handle of things.

Intermittent fasting is the way toward keeping a person's encouraging window constrained to only a couple of hours every day. It is an eating pattern that includes exchanging periods of eating and afterward, not eating by any stretch of the imagination.

Adopters of this method of planned eating have raved at its benefits, not the least of which is quick and huge weight misfortune, just as an expansion in vitality levels.

While superficially, it might appear as though it's unrealistic, the fact of the matter is intermittent fasting truly works. However, it's so well-known right now that there are heaps of clashing certainties and feelings gliding around in the open.

Typically, it won't abandon its myths, as most radical new thoughts will, in general, create. There are numerous regular misguided judgments concerning intermittent fasting, how about we attempt to expose a portion of those myths at this moment.

In case you need to try intermittent fasting out, however, are stressed over a portion of the things you've heard, it's smarter to adhere to certainties.

1) Your body will enter starvation mode

Basic thought directs that, on the off chance that you skip suppers, your body goes into starvation mode and begins to slow your digestion, believing that it is a "period of starvation." This has been the prevalent line of reasoning for quite a while, yet it's a legend.

The human body was intended to withstand the impacts of fasting as far back as we were cave dwellers.

Starvation is the point at which your muscle to fat ratio's stores are expended completely, so it must choose the option to separate tissue for vitality. This won't occur because you skipped breakfast.

With intermittent fasting, your body discharges put away fat and uses it as vitality, while your thin muscle tissue stays immaculate. This is particularly valid if you have a lot of fat stores effectively, which means your body has a ton to work with.

Ongoing contemplates on intermittent fasting additionally propose that fasting is useful to buy and significant health. Tests done on creatures that ate a rich diet of greasy foods in an eight-hour eating window and afterward fasted for the remainder of the day showed that they didn't get corpulent or show high insulin levels.

2) You can eat all you need in your eating window

This is perhaps the greatest fantasy encompassing intermittent fasting, and consequently, probably the most excellent trap for individuals who attempt intermittent fasting and battle with making it work. Because you've fasted for a specific measure of time and are presently in your eating window, it doesn't mean you can satrisfy your craves desire.

Getting thinner, even on intermittent fasting, is still about the caloric deficiency. It is highly unlikely you will lose weight if you surpass your support calories.

Contingent upon your age, tallness, weight, and muscle to fat ratio, there is a certain number of calories your body consumes for the day, mostly merely keeping up your present weight. On the off chance that you eat more than that number of calories during your eating window, at that point, you're going to put on weight regardless of how long you've fasted.

To keep yourself from gorging, it is ideal for screening your caloric admission. Besides, endeavor to eat a decent diet that incorporates a lot of products of the soil, and loads of fiber. Stay away from handled foods and foods that have a lot of additives. Stick to new, nutritious, and healthy food that is useful for your body.

3) You'll be ravenous constantly

Probably the greatest thing individuals stress over with intermittent fasting is that they could be eager always. It is a startling idea not to have the option to eat for 16 to 18 hours, or even as long as 20 hours every day. Individuals stress that they will be hungry each moment of consistently until they break their fast, which is a finished and complete fantasy.

Honestly, there is a "becoming accustomed to" period for intermittent fasting. First and foremost, you will experience food cravings that make you question what you're doing with your life. However, when your body acclimates to its new vitality utilization worldview, it will make changes to how your body works — including sentiments of appetite.

Intermittent fasting continuously becomes more straightforward as you slip yourself into it. Start by fasting for 14 hours every day for the initial two weeks, at that point knock your fasting window to 16 hours, until you're prepared for 18 (or remain at 16 hours if that works better for you). Keep in mind, tune in to your body and what it's attempting to let you know. You'll realize when you're prepared to kick it up an indent.

4) "It's an enchantment stunt."

While it might unquestionably feel like enchantment, given the speedy and unmistakable benefits, intermittent fasting is upheld by science, and numerous examinations have been done throughout the years to dissect its motivation and impacts. In spite of prevalent thinking, intermittent fasting isn't new. It's been around for a considerable length of time.

Generally, its study is essential — exhaust a larger number of calories than you are expending, and your body will be in a condition of caloric shortage. This will without a doubt, cause weight misfortune. Since 3,500 calories make up a pound, cutting 500 calories off your basal metabolic rate every day will guarantee you lose in any event one pound of weight securely every week.

What intermittent fasting additionally does is diminishes insulin levels during the fasting period, which betters encourage fat consuming.

In all actuality, intermittent fasting allows for progressively adaptable dietary patterns, which means you can eat a more significant amount of the food you appreciate as opposed to eating tasteless, bland, "healthy" food. Don't try too hard. Stick to great, nutritious food yet additionally, don't be reluctant to have a cut of cake now and then.

5) "It's simply one more trend/crash diet."

To expose this legend effectively, intermittent fasting isn't a diet, since it doesn't limit you from eating a specific food. In principle, you can eat a diet comprising of just pizza and brew, and you will lose weight as long as you keep up a caloric shortage.

This isn't prudent, as, in spite of the fact that you will lose weight, you won't be anyplace close to healthy with that sort of utilization. It's still better to adhere to a decent diet comprising of whole foods rich in protein, fiber, and nutrients. You can have a cut of pizza now and again, yet don't make it your staple.

Intermittent fasting is simply a guide on when you ought to eat, and when you ought not to eat. It's anything but a prevailing fashion or crash diet that guarantees mysterious body changes if you confine yourself from eating certain foods.

• PSYCHOLOGICAL BENEFITS

It's not astonishing then that intermittent fasting has developed as of late as one of the most utilized dietary techniques for supporting mental/intellectual health.

Intermittent fasting is another term for "time-confined eating," in which you eat just inside a specific "eating window." Researchers accept that intermittent fasting benefits both our cerebrums and bodies in a few different ways:

- The physiological impacts of willful fasting mirror those of starvation. Both intermittent fasting and food hardship are viewed as sorts of "positive stressors," simply as is work out. They cause the body to adjust in manners that advance health and battle infection, for example, by diminishing irritation, improving detoxification and upgrading cell reestablishment.

- Fasting has been shown to have hostile to maturing impacts in the human mind. It can help improve neuroplasticity (the cerebrum's capacity to frame new neural associations) and battle irritation, which connects to better memory, also enhanced the ability to learn and hold new data.

- Some studies have discovered that fasting can help bolster recuperation from cerebrum wounds and strokes and lower the risk for creating neurodegenerative sicknesses like Alzheimer's, dementia, and Parkinson's illness.

- Aside from its capacity to support psychological well-being, fasting likewise can help with disposition upgrade, weight misfortune/the board, counteractive action of diabetes, development of bulk, and substantially more.

Intermittent Fasting can be an amazingly successful method of shedding pounds, lessening irritation, and supercharging your mind. If you've been keeping awake to date on the most recent health and wellbeing patterns, presumably intermittent fasting has sprung up on your feed more than two or multiple times.

Intermittent fasting isn't another idea; in actuality, fasting has been used for health and life span for a considerable length of time. The health benefits of fasting are various and broad, particularly as more research has approved the benefits of intermittent fasting for weight misfortune as well as for some different parts of our health.

Probably the most amazing and energizing benefits of intermittent fasting are for our cerebrums. We should discuss our best 5 most loved benefits of intermittent fasting for your mind.

1. Lessens Inflammation

Intermittent fasting has been shown to altogether diminish irritation. Over the top aggravation is the reason for some ceaseless maladies that we face today, including Alzheimer's, dementia, obesity, diabetes, and then some. There are numerous methods for how intermittent fasting decreases aggravation.

- Autophagy — Autophagy is the point at which the body wrecks old or harmed cells. Consider it like wiping off the rust and purifying itself. It's a method for the body fixing itself. On the off chance that old or harmed cells stay in the body, they make aggravation. Intermittent fasting invigorates autophagy, helping the body to purge itself, in this manner decreasing irritation

- Ketones — The body uses up the ketones during fasting and every last bit of its sugar stores and needs to go to fat for fuel. At the point when fats get separated, it makes ketones. One of the most plentiful ketones, β-hydroxybutyrate, really squares some portion of the invulnerable framework liable for controlling fiery issues like joint pain and even Alzheimers.

- Insulin Sensitive — Fasting has been shown to help settle insulin opposition. At the point when the body gets impervious to insulin, insulin and glucose develop in the blood and make aggravation. Intermittent fasting permits your body to take a break. Since there is no food to process and your body uses up the entirety of its sugar stores, insulin levels start to drop, allowing the body to re-sharpen to insulin once more.

2. Make More Brain Cells

Truly! You can make more synapses and in this manner, improve your intellectual competence. Fasting has been shown to expand paces of neurogenesis in the cerebrum. Neurogenesis is the development and improvement of new synapses and nerve tissues.

3. Lift "Supernatural occurrence Grow" In Your Brain

In addition to the fact that fasting increases your pace of neurogenesis, it likewise helps the generation of a significant protein called BDNF. BDNF has been hailed as "Marvel Grow For Your Brain."

BDNF has been shown to assume a job in neuroplasticity, which allows the mind to proceed to change and adjust. It makes your cerebrum stronger to stress and increasingly versatile to adapt.

BDNF creates new synapses, secures your synapses, animates new associations, and neural connections while additionally boosting memory, improving the state of mind, and learning.

Intermittent fasting has been shown to support BDNF by 50–400%.

4. Consumes Fat for Fuel Instead Of Sugar

This may come as a stun, yet fat is a superior and cleaner wellspring of fuel than starches. In addition to the fact that fat produces more vitality per gram than starches do. However, it creates less free radicals, which cause aggravation. When your mitochondria, your cells batteries, utilize fat (ketones) or starches to make vitality, there is squander that gets as free radicals.

Free radicals cause oxidative worry to the body and are believed to be the reason for some interminable maladies we face today, including numerous neurodegenerative illnesses.

Intermittent fasting powers your cerebrum to utilize ketones, as opposed to sugar, which is cleaner and increasingly proficient fuel for your mind.

5. Lifts Human Growth Hormone

Upon first hearing human development hormone (HGH), you may have an image of a weight lifter utilizing it to get gigantic muscles. HGH from an exogenous source (all things considered) isn't prescribed for a wide assortment of reasons and isn't the best for your body.

HGH has been found to have a fantastically amazing enemy of maturing and life span benefits, however accurately, HGH can improve comprehension, give neuroprotection, and increment neurogenesis.

The HGH had a neuroprotective impact, safeguarding your mental health and cerebrum execution.

Intermittent fasting has been shown to regularly support HGH levels to give healthy hostile to maturing, fix, neuroprotective, and life span benefits.

6. Supercharges Your Energy

Intermittent Fasting has been shown to support mitochondrial biogenesis, the production of new mitochondria. As we've referenced before, mitochondria are the batteries for your cells. Every last one of your cells is loaded up with many mitochondria that power your cells to carry out their responsibility. Their main responsibility is to take the food you eat and transform it into vitality.

• USEFUL RECIPES FOR INTERMITTENT FASTING

Although "fasting" sounds alarming, intermittent fasting (IF) is overwhelming the diet world. On the diet's positive effect on body weight, insight, and glucose, it's no big surprise that everybody you know is by all accounts getting on board with the IF fleeting trend. Perhaps the intrigue is the absence of food rules. There are limitations on when you can eat, yet not really what you can eat. So would it be a good idea for you to down pints of frozen yogurt and packs of chips while intermittent fasting? Likely not. That is the reason we've concocted a rundown of the best foods to incorporate into your IF life.

Intermittent Fasting Refresher

There are multiple IF plans, yet most spotlight on fasting for a specific number of hours in the days of the week. Here's a breakdown of the most famous IF models.

12:12 Method

Fast for 12 hours every day and eat inside a 12-hour window. In the event that you eat your last feast at 7 p.m. furthermore, eat the following morning at 7 a.m., congrats, you're now an IF expert. (This is useful for amateurs.)

20:4 Method

Fast for an entire 20 hours and allow yourself one four-hour window to eat.

16:8 Method

Eat your day by day food inside an 8-hour window and fast for the staying 16 hours.

5:2 Method

Eat anything you desire for 5 days out of the week. For the other two days, men can expend 600 calories, while ladies can devour 500 calories.

So WTF Should I Eat?

"There are no determinations or limitations about what type or how much food to eat while following intermittent fasting. Be that as it may, "the benefits [of IF] are not liable to go with reliable suppers.

A well-adjusted diet is a way to shedding pounds, keeping up vitality levels, and staying with the diet. "Anybody endeavoring to lose weight should concentrate on nutrient-thick foods, similar to organic products, veggies, entire grains, nuts, beans, seeds, just as dairy and fit proteins.

1. Water

Although you aren't eating, it's essential to remain hydrated for such a significant number of reasons, similar to the health of fundamentally every significant organ in your body. The measure of water that any one individual should drink changes, yet you need your pee to be a light yellow shading consistently. Dull yellow pee demonstrates a lack of hydration, which can cause cerebral pains, exhaustion, and discombobulation. Couple that with constrained food, and it could be a catastrophe waiting to happen. If the idea of plain water doesn't energize you, include a crush of a lemon squeeze, a couple of mint leaves, or cucumber cuts to your water. It'll be our little mystery.

2. Avocado

It might appear to be outlandish to eat the most unhealthy organic product while attempting to lose weight, yet the monounsaturated fat in avocado is amazingly satisfying. Including a portion of an avocado to your lunch may keep you full for a considerable length of time longer than if you didn't eat the green jewel.

3. Fish

There's an explanation the Dietary Guidelines propose eating, in any event, eight ounces of fish every week. If it is rich in healthy fats and protein, it likewise contains adequate measures of nutrient D. What's more, in case you're just eating a constrained measure of food for the day, don't you need one that conveys nutrient-value progressively for your money? Also that restricting your calorie admission may upset your comprehension, and fish is frequently viewed as a mind food.

4. Cruciferous and Veggies

Diets like broccoli, Brussels sprouts, and cauliflower are on the whole brimming with the f-word—fiber. At the point when you're eating inconsistently, it's essential to eat fiber-rich foods that will keep you customary and avert constipation. Fiber likewise can make you feel full, which is something you may need on the off chance that you can't eat again for 16 hours.

5. Potatoes

Rehash after me: Not every single white food is awful. A valid example: Studies have seen potatoes as one of the most satisfying foods around. Another study found that eating vegetables as a component of a healthy diet could help with weight misfortune. Apologies, French fries, and potato chips don't tally.

5. Beans and Legumes

Your preferred expansion to stew might be your closest companion on the IF way of life. Food, explicitly carbs, supplies vitality for movement. While we're not guiding you to carbo-load, it certainly wouldn't damage to toss some low-calorie carbs, similar to beans and vegetables, into your eating plan. Also, foods like chickpeas, dark berries, peas, and lentils have been shown to diminish body weight, even without calorie limitation.

6. The Pro-biotics

Consistency and decent variety that implies they are disturbed when they're ravenous. What's more, when your gut is upset, you may encounter some disturbing symptoms, similar to constipation. To check this obnoxiousness, include probiotic-rich foods, like kefir, a fermented tea, or kraut, to your diet.

7. Berries

Your preferred smoothie expansion is ready with essential nutrients. Strawberries are an extraordinary wellspring of invulnerable boosting nutrient C, with more than 100 percent of the everyday esteem in one cup. What's more, that is not by any means the best part—individuals who devoured a diet rich in flavonoids, similar to those in blueberries and strawberries, had littler increments in BMI over 14 years than the individuals who didn't eat berries.

8. Eggs

One enormous egg has six grams of protein and concocts in minutes. Getting, however much protein, as could be expected, is significant for keeping full and building muscle. Men who had an egg breakfast rather than a bagel were less hungry and ate less for the day. At the dawn of the day, when you're searching for something to do during your fasting period, why not hard-heat up certain eggs?

9. Nuts

They might be higher in calories than numerous different bites, yet nuts contain something that most lousy nourishment doesn't—high fat. Polyunsaturated fat in pecans can modify the physiological markers for appetite and satiety.

Furthermore, in case you're stressed over calories, don't be! A one-ounce serving of almonds (around 23 nuts) has 20 percent fewer calories than recorded on the name. Fundamentally, the biting procedure doesn't separate the almond cell dividers, leaving a bit of the nut unblemished and unabsorbed during assimilation.

10. Entire Grains

Being on a diet and eating carbs appear as though they have a place in two distinct pails, yet not generally! Whole grains are nutritious in fiber and protein, therefore eating a little goes far in keeping you full. Besides, Eating entire grains rather than refined grains may really fire up your digestion. So feel free to eat your entire grains and adventure out of your usual range of familiarity to attempt farro, bulgur, spelled, Kamut, amaranth, millet, sorghum, or freekeh.

Low-Calorie recipes for the Intermittent Fasting Plan

The 5:2 Method And Intermittent Fasting.

The Intermittent Fasting otherwise the 5:2 diet, was concocted about the impacts of fasting on the human body. The human system benefits from periods of intermittent fasting and that a portion of those benefits incorporates practical weight misfortune, lowered levels of blood cholesterol, a decrease in the risk of malignant growth, cardiovascular sickness, and Alzheimer's.

Intermittent fasting is the way toward switching back and forth between periods of fasting, where caloric admission is severely confined, and periods of 'devouring' where caloric admission isn't limited.

Ladies ought to yield to the consumption of 600 calories on fasting days and 700 calories for men. On non-fasting days, you can adhere to your typical diet.

Many people attempting to lose weight needs to yield to a pattern of two days of fasting for particular week, and five days of non-fasting (ie. healthy eating) are most effectively attainable and viable. It is significant however not to indulge on non-fasting days and to adhere to a systematic eating pattern and diet. If you find that your weight misfortune has slowed down, you can modify the method to a 4:3 method, where you fast for three days and blowout for 4 days per week. When you have arrived at your actual weight, a 6:1 pattern can be followed to keep up your weight.

By following the 5:2 diet, a great many people can hope to lose somewhere in the range of one and two pounds each week.

About the Recipes

Every one of the plans is anything but difficult to adjust to your taste.

Adjusting the Recipes to Suit You

The entirety of the plans in this book is genuinely versatile. On the off chance that you change any of the fixings, however, it's critical even now to know what number calories you are eating, so you should discover the measure of calories per standard of food you are eating.

Coconut Oil

Any coconut oil will do. On the off chance that it's healthy, but the container in high temp water to allow it to melt. The liver handles coconut oil as opposed to it being put away as fat like such a large number of different sorts of oils.

If you don't mind the flavor of coconut, utilize refined coconut oil as opposed to virgin coconut oil.

Ten grams of coconut oil contain around 90 calories, so on your fasting day, you could make due on only 5 serves of coconut oil.

I put it in unsweetened espresso to make what is known as slug verification espresso.

Different methods for eating coconut oil:

- In low-calorie yogurt
- Swallow it straight (not my thing but rather a few people may have the option to do it)
- Mixed with a fried egg
- On plates of mixed greens
- Ideal for broiling as it has an exceptionally high smoke point (particularly refined coconut oil)
- In sauces

Yogurt, Berries, and Pepitas

This is a flavorful sweet, filling dish that is high in protein and different minerals and nutrients yet low in calories, so you could stand to eat it 2-3 times on a fasting day or to have a bigger sum in one sitting.

100g Unsweetened regular yogurt = 84 calories

100g mixed berries (I like to crush mine in my Nutri-projectile) = 43 calories

10g Pepitas = 50 calories

Stevia to taste = 0 Calories

Complete calories: 177

Yogurt, Berries, and Pepitas

Home-made Coconut And Banana Ice Cream

Fish and Mustard on Toast

- 70g jar of fish (you may wish to utilize salmon, trout or sardines) with spring water rather than oil = around 80 calories
- 1 cut of bread = 72.5 calories (using 'Has No' sans gluten bread)
- 10 g of whole grain french mustard = around 15 calories
- Total calories = around 162.5 calories

Stuffed Mushrooms

This dish is one for mushroom darlings. Calories will fluctuate contingent upon the fixings and brands utilized; however, for mine, I tallied 359 calories.

Utilize:

- 3 medium Portobello mushrooms - 250g = 55 calories
- Low-fat ricotta cheddar - 100g = 116 calories
- Low-fat ground cheddar cheddar - 40g = 130 calories
- Boneless leg ham 40g = 45 calories
- Chopped parsley - 1/4 cup = 6 calories
- Dice red capsicum - 30g = 8 calories

Readiness:

- Pre-heat stove to 180 degrees Celsius
- Remove the stems from the mushrooms and shakers them
- Finely cut the ham
- Combine the ham, capsicum, parsley, ricotta cheddar and diced mushroom stems in a bowl and blend well
- Spoon the above blend into the rearranged mushrooms
- Sprinkle with the ground cheddar
- Cook in pre-warmed stove still at 180 degrees Celsius for 20 minutes

Rice Cakes, Banana And Nutella

A thinny smear of Nutella on two rice cake, bested with a little meagerly cut banana, with some skim milk.

Around 200 calories altogether.

A Bowl Of Popcorn.

25g of air-popped popping corn = 91 calories

Cooked in 5ml of oil include around 50 calories = around 141 calories

Mushroom Delight

Mushrooms are exceptionally low in calories yet very filling.

- 260g cleaved Portobello mushrooms
- 75g cleaved green beans
- 50g ground zucchini
- 1 spring onion
- 2 enormous eggs (90g each)
- 5g minced garlic
- 10g wholegrain mustard
- 10g ground cheddar

1. Mix all fixings with the exception of cheddar and eggs in a non-stick skillet and cook for 5 to 10 minutes on heating (no oil is required as the mushrooms will lose water which will flow into the griddle).
2. Include eggs and cook for a further 1-2 minutes
3. Remove from warmth and present with cheddar sprinkled on top

All out calories: around 270.

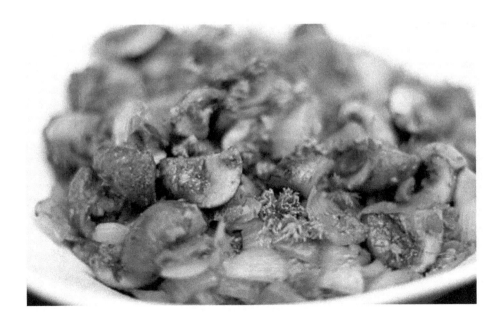

Kiwi And Red Capsicum

This is a flavorful tidbit low in calories and high in Vitamin C and enemies of oxidants.

Cut one kiwi natural product (100g = 20 calories) and some red capsicum (100g = 40 calories).

Red capsicum is additionally known as a red ringer pepper.

Letttuce Leaf Wrap

- 2 leaf of Cos lettuce - 8 calories
- 25g ground crude carrot - 9 calories
- 25g ground zucchini - 4 calories
- 50g cut chicken bosom - 83 calories

Complete calories: 104 calories

Carrot And Capsicum Snack

In case you're feeling somewhat peckish between dinners on your fasting days, you should attempt this nibble of ground carrot with cleaved crude capsicum (otherwise called ringer pepper). Calories will shift contingent upon the sum you eat. However, this is an exceptionally low-calorie nibble. Utilize the MyFitnessPal application to check the number of calories you're expending.

Chicken Salad

Counting some quality protein in your dinners will help keep you feeling full for more.

This formula requires a chicken patty with a vegetable serving of mixed greens.

Chicken burger - Woolworths Select brand - 125g = 181 caloroes

Rice Cake Treat

A low calorie with high protein filling nibble, or have a few for a dinner.

- One rice cake - calories change by the brand yet around 25 - 46 calories
- 3 grape tomatoes - 4 calories
- 1/2 teaspoon Basil and garlic mince - homemade utilizing a mortar and pestle - 3 calories
- 1 tablespoon of low-fat curds - around 15 calories

All out calories: 47-67 calories for every serve.

Green Smoothie

A green smoothie is an ideal method to guarantee you're getting a healthy serve of greens. Mix some verdant green vegetables with a large portion of some skim milk. If you care not for the flavor of just greens, add some natural product however attempt to adhere to only one bit of organic product to downplay the caloric burden.

- 1/2 cup of skim milk = 45 calories
- 1 Valencia orange = 85 calories or 1 little ready banana = 90 calories
- 1 cup of slashed verdant green vegetables, for example, kale, spinach, chard, Pak Choy = 50 calories

All out calories = 185

Low-Calorie Carbonara

Slendier noodles are very filling and nutritious; however, best of all, they contain just 8 calories for every 100 grams!!

For this formula I utilized:

- 250g bundle of Slendier noodles (20 calories)
- 160mls low-fat thickened cream,
- Bacon with the fat expelled,
- parmesan cheddar to taste,
- rice grain cooking splash to cook the bacon.

Directions:

1. Cut bacon into a little pieces and fry it in a cooking splash or a minimum quantity of cooking oil
2. Add thickened cream and leave to bubble for a few minutes to make the sauce
3. Remove sauce from heat
4. Prepare noodles according to guidelines on bundle
5. Add sauce to noodles and combine
6. Add parmesan cheddar to taste, however, make certain to quantify how a lot of you're including so you can work out what number calories are in it.
7. Cook noodles according to directions on the bundle

Gauge your fixings first to work out the measure of calories in this tasty dish. For me, it signified 330 Calories.

Clear Mushroom Soup

Fixings:

- Thick Portabello, Field, and Shitake mushrooms (enough to fulfill).
- Two cloves garlic.
- Five cut shallots.
- Two little chillis.
- Two spring onions, slight cut.

Method:

- Lightly fry in a deep pot with a little shower of oil
- Add 500 ml of Chicken, Beef, or instead Vegetable stock.
- Ground pepper to taste.
- Bring to a bubble, at that point stew 20 mins or as wanted.
- This supper is more often than not around 100 calories relying upon amounts.

Cauliflower-outside layer pizza

This is pizza-darling's 5:2 method for eating pizza. The base is a lot of lower in calories and starches than wheat-based pizza bases, so it's a perfect option in contrast to conventional pizza-batter.

There are loads of various plans for making cauliflower-outside pizza, and below, you'll see a video for the formula that functions admirably for me.

Include your low-calorie fixings - I ordinarily include mushrooms, shaved low-fat ham or shaved turkey bosom, ground zucchini, onions, and low-fat ground cheddar.

The complete calories will rely upon the garnishes utilized and the fixings in the base.

Crushed Cauliflower

Crushed cauliflower is a low-calorie, low-sugar, and more delicious option to pureed potatoes. Essentially steam some cauliflower at that point squash it.

Include a touch of garlic, some low-fat ricotta cheddar or curds for protein and calcium, a run of Parmesan cheddar, and a spot of salt.

RED CABBAGE AND GREEN APPLE SESAME SLAW

Serves 2

Fixings

For the plate of blended greens:

3 cups daintily obliterated red cabbage

1 colossal granny smith apple, devastated

2 table spoon hemp seeds

For the dressing:

1/4 cup tahini

3 tablespoons water

2 teaspoons agave nectar or maple syrup

1/2 teaspoon sesame oil

1/4 – 1/2 tsp of sea salt (to taste)

1 tablespoon squeezed apple vinegar

Procedure

1. Whisk dressing fixings together and put in a sheltered spot.

2. Dress the wrecked vegetables and hemp seeds with dressing; you can use as much as you can envision, however, guarantee you coat everything incredible (a half-cup will probably take care of business). Serve. Slaw will keep in the cooler medium-term.

Fixings

For the serving of blended greens:

5 cups washed, dried, and sliced kale (around 1 group after planning)

2 little carrots, ground

2 stalk celery, sliced

4 table spoon splendid raisins

4 table spoon sliced walnuts

1 apple, cut pitiful

For the dressing:

2 table spoon olive oil

1/2 table spoon squeezed apple

1 table spoon agave

Salt and pepper to taste

Strategy

1. Whisk the dressing fixings together, and put in a protected spot.

2. In a huge mixing bowl, pour about the dressing onto the sliced kale and start "scouring"

3. Plate the serving of blended greens and top it with your cut apple. Appreciate. Remains will keep medium-term in the fridge.

SMOKY AVOCADO AND JICAMA SALAD

Fixings

For the dressing:

One minimal avocado

1 table spoon cumin powder

Juice of 2 limes

1/2 teaspoon smoked paprika

1 cup of water

1/4 tsp salt

Run cayenne pepper

For the plate of blended greens:

1 heaping cup devastated cabbage

1 heaping cup devastated carrot

10 immense leaves romaine lettuce, cut pitifully

2 cups jicama, cut into matchsticks

2 table spoon toasted pumpkin seeds

Methodology

1. Mix all dressing fixings in a blender or processor till smooth.

2. Pour dressing over this plate of blended greens, and fling. Serve.

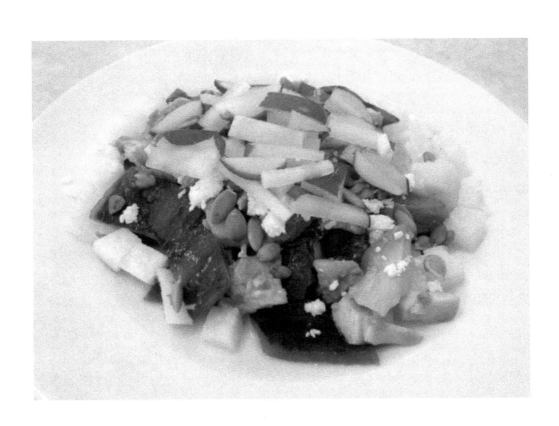

MANGO, KALE, AND AVOCADO SALAD
Serves 2

Fixings:

1 pack wavy kale, de-stemmed, cut, washed, and dried (around 6 cups after readiness)

Juice of 1 colossal lemon

2 teaspoons flax or olive oil

1 teaspoon sesame oil

2 teaspoons maple syrup or agave nectar

Sea salt to taste.

1 hacked red ringer pepper

1 cup mango, cut into little 3D squares

1 little Haas avocado, cut into 3D squares

System

1. "Backrub" the lemon juice, flax/olive and sesame oils, syrup, and salt into the kale till it's dried and dressed impartially.

2. Blend in the pepper, mango, and avocado 3D squares. Throw well to join. Serve.

STEWED BUTTERNUT SQUASH AND APPLE SOUP

Makes 4 servings

Fixings

1 butternut squash, stripped and hacked (around 3-4 lbs, or 4-5 cups)

3 little apples, by and large hacked

1 little onion, hacked

2 table spoon disintegrated coconut oil

1/2 tsp authentic or sea salt (+more to taste)

Dim pepper to taste

1/4 tsp nutmeg

1/2 tsp squashed thyme

2 1/2 cups low sodium vegetable soup

1/2 cup canned coconut milk

Methodology

1. Spot squash, apples, and onion on a large stewing plate. Sprinkle coconut oil and salt and pepper over them, mix with your hands, and dish at 375 degrees for 45 minutes, or until they're all sensitive and splendid.

2. Spot cooked veggies in a blender with vegetable stock, nutmeg, coconut milk, and thyme. If the soup needs dynamically liquid, incorporate some more until it lands at the consistency you like.

3. Move soup to a pot, re-warmth, and serve.

CURRIED YELLOW LENTILS WITH AVOCADO "Bread trims."

Serves 4

Fixings

3/4 cup onion, diced

1/2 table spoon coconut oil

1 cup yellow lentils

1 bowl of sweet potato, cut into 1/2 inch 3D shapes

2 carrots, diced (optional, yet I had them, so I used them!)

1/2 tsp turmeric

1 table spoon delicate curry powder

1 tsp powdered ginger

1/2 tsp sea salt

Dull pepper to taste

4 cups vegetable soup or water

Technique

1. Heat the oil in a huge pot over medium warmth. Saute onion till its turning translucent and to some degree splendid. Incorporate the lentils, potato, carrots, and flavors/seasonings, and mix to solidify everything.

2. Add the juices or water to the pot and warmth to the point of bubbling. Lessen to a stew and cook for 25 minutes, or until the lentils and sweet potato are sensitive.

3. Allow lentils to cool to some degree, by then present with new avocado cuts.

KALE SALAD, APPLES, RAISINS, WITH CARROTS, AND CREAMY CURRY DRESSING

Serves 2-4

Fixings

For the dressing:

1/2 cup rough cashews or walnuts

2 tablespoons lemon juice

2 set dates

1/2 cup water

1/2 tsp sea salt

2 tsp curry powder

For the plate of blended greens:

1 head kale, de-stemmed, washed, dried, and chop into downsized pieces (around 5 cups)

2 gigantic carrots, stripped and hacked

1 gigantic apple, hacked into little pieces

1/3 cup raisins

1/2 cup chickpeas

System

1. Mix all dressing fixings in a fast blender till smooth.

2. Back rub the kale with the dressing, guaranteeing that everything is all around secured and mellowed (start with 1/2 cup dressing and incorporate as required—you may make them remain). Incorporate the apple, carrot, raisins, and chickpeas, and remix the serving of blended greens, including all the more dressing in case you like. Serve.

RED QUINOA, ALMOND AND ARUGULA SALAD WITH CANTALOUPE

Makes 2 servings

Fixings

1/2 cups fresh melon, cut into 1-inch pieces

1/2 cups red quinoa (standard quinoa is also totally lovely)

4 cups arugula, immovably squeezed

1/4 cup divided, deteriorated, or cut almonds

2 tablespoons flax, hemp, or olive oil

1 tablespoon squeezed apple vinegar

2

1 teaspoon maple syrup

Sea salt and dull pepper to taste

Technique

1. Whisk together the oil, vinegar, syrup, and seasoning.

2. Separation the arugula, quinoa, and melon onto two serving plates. Sprinkle them with almonds and a while later shower the dressing over them.

HOT THAI SALAD

Serves 2

Fixings

For the dressing:

1 avocado

1 cup of coconut water

¼ cup cilantro

¼ cup basil

¼ tsp salt (or continuously) 2 set dates

1 table spoon minced or ground ginger Sprinkle of cayenne pepper

For the plate of blended greens:

1 toll pepper, sliced

2 cups ground carrots

1/2 cup cilantro, hacked

1 cup develops

2 cups annihilated romaine lettuce

1 cup cut cucumbers

Technique

1. Mix all dressing fixings in a quick blender till smooth.

2. The top plate of blended greens in with dressing as needed. Serve.

CARROT AVOCADO BISQUE

Serves 2

Fixings

2 cups carrot juice

1/2 Haas avocado

1 tablespoon low sodium tamari

1 teaspoon ground ginger

Technique

Blend all fixings in a quick blender till smooth.

GLUTEN-FREE TORTILLA PIZZA

Serves 2

Fixings

2 10" darker rice tortillas (Food for Life brand)

2/3 cup low sodium, characteristic marinara sauce, separated

2 cups vegetable + trimmings of choice (broccoli, spinach, peppers, mushrooms, olives, artichokes, cooked potato, etc.)

1/2 cup crucial cashew cheddar (equation underneath)

Strategy

1. Preheat flame broil to 400 F. Spot tortillas on a foil or material lined warming sheet. Plan for 5-

8 minutes, or until hardly new.

2. Expel tortillas from oven, and return to the barbecue for 8-

10 additional minutes (till enhancements are cooked through). The bit with cashew cheddar, and serve.

NB: If you don't have cashew cheddar, you can sprinkle pizzas with feeding yeast.

You can similarly use red pepper hummus rather than the tomato sauce.

CASHEW CHEESE

Makes 1 cup

Fixings

1/4 cups cashews, sprinkled for in any occasion three hours (or medium-term) and exhausted 1/2 tsp sea salt

1 little clove garlic, minced (optional)

2 table spoon lemon juice

1/3-1/2 cup water

1/4 cup sustaining yeast

Strategy

Recognize the cashews, sea salt, garlic, lemon, and 1/3 cup water in a sustenance processor. Methodology till the mix is particularly smooth and fragile (you're going for a surface like smooth ricotta cheddar), stopping to scratch the bowl down a few times and including some extra water as fundamental.

COOKED CAULIFLOWER AND PARSNIP SOUP

Yields 4 servings

Fixings

1 medium head cauliflower, separated

4 gigantic parsnips, stripped and sliced

1-2 table spoon olive oil

4 shallots, chop down the center

1 clove garlic, minced

1 tsp thyme

1/2 tsp sage

4 cups vegetable stock

1/2 cup almond or coconut milk

Sea salt and pepper to taste

Paprika

Technique

1. Preheat stove to 400 degrees. Line a getting ready plate or two with tin foil.

2. Lay cauliflower, parsnips, shallots, and garlic, out on foil, and shower with olive oil, thyme, wine, salt and pepper.

3. Broil veggies for around 35-40 min, or until they're fragile and splendid dull shaded.

4. Spot veggies in a quick blender (you may need to work in gatherings) and incorporate stock and non-dairy milk. Blend until the soup is smooth and rich, including logically liquid in case you need to. Then again, you can use an immersion blender.

5. Move soup to a pot and re-season to taste with salt and pepper.

Tidbits

HEMP HUMMUS

Serves 4

Fixings

1/4 cup shelled hemp seeds

1 can chickpeas, exhausted, or 2 cups recently cooked chickpeas 1/2 tsp salt (to taste)

2-3 table spoon recently squeezed lemon juice (to taste)

1 little clove garlic, minced

1 table spoon tahini (optional)

1/2 tsp cumin

Water as required

System

1. Spot the hemp seeds in the bowl of a sustenance processor and grind till fine.

2. Include the chickpeas, salt, lemon, garlic, tahini, and cumin, and begin to process. Incorporate water in a slight stream (stopping to scratch the bowl a few times) until the mix is completely smooth and smooth.

3. Trimming with extra hemp seeds and serve.

Nutty spread AND JELLY SNACK BALLS

Makes 20 Balls

Fixings

1/2 cups characteristic seared, unsalted peanuts

1/2 cups dull raisins

2 tablespoons nutty spread

Press sea salt

Technique

1. Add all fixings to a sustenance processor and method till the peanuts are isolated and the mix is starting to stay together. It may release a little oil. However, that is OK.

2. Fold mix into 1 inch balls. Store in the fridge for on any occasion thirty minutes before serving.

SWEET POTATO HUMMUS

Serves 6

Fixings

2 cups sweet potato, steamed or warmed and cut into 3D shapes

1 can regular, low sodium chickpeas, drained (or 1/2 cups cooked chickpeas)

1/2 tsp sesame oil

1/4 cup tahini

1 tablespoon lemon juice

1/2 tsp smoked paprika

1/2 tsp salt

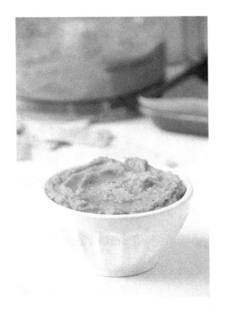

TURMERIC TAHINI DRESSING

Makes 1/2 Cups

Fixings

1/2 cup tahini

2 tablespoons squeezed apple vinegar

2 tablespoons coconut aminos or tamari

1/2 teaspoonful of ginger (or 1 teaspoon fresh, ground ginger)

2 teaspoons turmeric

1 teaspoon maple syrup

2/3 - 3/4 cup water

Procedure

Mix all the fixings in a blender till smooth. Start with 2/3 cup water and incorporate more as required (dressing will thicken in the cooler).

Walnut PESTO

Makes 1 liberal cup

Fixings

1 cup coarsely sliced walnuts

2 1/2 cups squeezed new basil leaves, washed and dried

1 huge garlic clove

1 table spoon lemon style

Juice of 1 lemon

1/4 cup healthy yeast

1/2 cup high extra virgin olive oil

Salt and pepper to taste

Procedure

1. Crush walnuts in a sustenance processor till finely ground. Incorporate basil and heartbeat till it outlines a rough mix.

2. Include the garlic, lemon style and squeeze, and dietary yeast, and heartbeat a few additional events. Turn the motor on and continue running as you incorporate olive oil in a meager stream. I like my pesto outstandingly thick, however, combine more oil if you need an increasingly thin mix. Add salt and pepper to taste. Use, or stop as required.

BALSAMIC TAHINI DRESSING

Makes 1/4 cups

Fixings

1/2 cup tahini

1/4 cup balsamic vinegar

1/2 cup water

1/4 teaspoon of garlic powder, or 1/2 clove finely minced garlic 1 table spoon tamari or nama shoyu

Technique

Grind all fixings in a blender. Incorporate more water as required.

Unrefined RANCH DRESSING

Makes 1 ½ cups

Fixings

¾ cup cashews, soaked for in any occasion two hours and exhausted ½ cup water

2 table spoon lemon juice

¼ cup squeezed apple vinegar ¼-½ teaspoon salt.

½ tsp dried thyme ½ tsp dried oregano 1 clove garlic

3 table spoon new dill

3 table spoon new parsley

3 table spoon olive oil

System

Blend all fixings in a fast blender and serve.

SMOOTH APRICOT GINGER DRESSING

Makes around 2 cups (equation can be separated)

Fixings

1/2 cup dried apricots, stuffed

3/4 inch long handle rough ginger (or 1/2 tsp ginger powder)

1/2 cup crushed orange

1/2 cup water

2 table spoon squeezed apple vinegar

1 table spoon tamari or nama shoyu

2 table spoon olive oil

Methodology

Blend all dressing fixings in a fast blender and serve.

Fig and White Balsamic Vinaigrette

Makes 1/4 cups

Fixings

6 extraordinarily immense dried figs (if yours are pretty much nothing, incorporate several inexorably), soaked for around 8 hours and exhausted

1/3 white balsamic vinegar (subordinary if need be)

1/4 cup olive oil

1/4 water

1 little clove garlic

1 table spoon dijon mustard

Salt and dull pepper to taste

Strategy

Blend all fixings in an electric blender till totally smooth and velvety. Incorporate more water if it's unnecessarily thick.

Dim BEAN AND QUINOA SALAD WITH QUICK CUMIN DRESSING

Serves 4

Fixings

For the serving of blended greens:

1 cup dry quinoa, flushed

Run salt

2 cups vegetable squeezes or water

1/2 colossal cucumber, diced perfectly

1 little ringer pepper, diced immaculately

1 can BPA free, regular dull beans

10-15 basil leaves, hacked into a chiffonade

1/4 cup new cilantro, hacked

For the vinaigrette:

2 table spoon extra virgin olive oil

1/4 cup squeezed apple vinegar

1 table spoon agave or maple syrup

1 table spoon dijon mustard

1 tsp cumin

Salt and pepper to taste

System

1. Flush quinoa through a strainer till the water runs clear. Move it to a little or medium evaluated pot and incorporate two cups of vegetable squeezes or water and run of salt. Spread the bowl with the objective that the top is on, yet there's a little gap where water can escape. Stew till quinoa has ingested most of the liquid and is fluffy (around 15-20 minutes).

2. Move cooked quinoa to a mixing bowl. Incorporate divided vegetables, dim beans, and herbs.

3. Whisk dressing fixings. Add the dressing to the plate of blended greens, and serve.

1) Serving of blended greens will keep for three days in the cooler.

ZUCCHINI PASTA WITH, BASIL, SWEET POTATO, HEMP PARMESAN, AND CHERRY TOMATOES

Serves 2

Fixings

2 colossal zucchini

1 red ringer pepper, diced

15 cherry tomatoes, quartered

8 colossal basil leaves, chiffonaded

2 minimal sweet potato, warmed and after that cut into strong shapes

2 table spoon balsamic vinegar

1 minimal avocado, cubed

4 table spoon hemp parmesan (equation underneath)

Procedure

1. Utilize the spiralizer to cut zucchini into long strips (looking like noodles).

2. Hurl zucchini with every lingering fixing, and serve.

Hemp Parmesan

Makes 1/2 - 2/3 cup

Fixings

6 table spoon hemp seeds

6 table spoon supporting yeast

Run sea salt

Procedure

Join all fixings in a sustenance processor, and heartbeat to isolate and unite. Store in the icebox for whatever length of time that around fourteen days.

GLUTEN-FREE WHITE BEAN AND SUMMER VEGETABLE PASTA

Serves 4

Fixings

1 little eggplant, cut into 1-inch 3D squares and tenderly salted for 30 minutes, by then tap dry

1 clove garlic, minced

1 would naturally have the option to fire stewed, diced tomatoes

1 little can regular tomato sauce

1 tsp agave

1 table spoon dried basil

1 tsp dried oregano

1 tsp dried thyme

1 can (or 2 cups recently cooked) cannellini or maritime power beans, exhausted

8 oz. dry dim hued rice or quinoa pasta (rigatoni, linguine, and penne are all in all fine)

System

1. Warmth a deep skillet with olive or coconut oil shower (or use a few table spoon glasses of water).

2. Include the zucchini and cook it till sensitive.

3. Incorporate the canned tomatoes, agave, basil, oregano, tomato sauce, thyme. Warmth through. Test for enhancing, and incorporate a higher measure of whatever herbs you like.

4. Include the white beans and warmth the whole sauce through. This is so heavenly and essential, and you could eat it in solitude as "con artist.

5. At the point when your sauce is cooking, put a pot of salted water to bubble. Incorporate pasta when it hits a moving air pocket, and cook pasta till fragile yet simultaneously to some degree still to some degree firm.

6. Channel pasta, spread with sauce and serve.

Remains will keep for three days in the cooler.

BUTTERNUT SQUASH CURRY

Serves 4

Fixings

1 tablespoon broke up coconut oil

1 white or yellow onion, hacked

1 clove garlic, minced

1 tablespoon new ginger, minced

3 tablespoons red curry stick

1 tablespoon regular sugar or coconut sugar

2/3 cups vegetable soup

One 14-or 15-ounce would coconut have the option to deplete.

One green or red ringer pepper, hacked.

2-pound butternut squash

1 cups green beans, cut into 2" pieces

1 to 2 tablespoon lime juice

Strategy

1. Warmth the coconut oil in a huge pot or wok. Incorporate the onion and cook till it's fragile and translucent (5 to 8 minutes).

2. Blend the garlic and ginger, let them cook for about a minute. By then, incorporate the curry paste and sugar. Join the fixings until the paste is evenhandedly melded.

3. Race in the juices, the coconut milk, and the tamari. Incorporate the red pepper and butternut squash. Stew till the squash is sensitive (25 to 30 minutes). If you need to incorporate extra stock as the mix cooks, do like this.

4. Blend the green beans and let them cook for a couple of moments, or until sensitive. Add the curry to taste with extra soy sauce or tamari and blend in the lime press as needed. Remove from warmth and serve over quinoa or dim shaded basmati rice.

Remains will keep for four days.

Rough ZUCCHINI ALFREDO WITH BASIL AND CHERRY TOMATOES

Serves 2 (with remaining alfredo sauce)

Fixings

Pasta

Two tremendous zucchini

1 cup cherry tomatoes, split

1/4 cup basil, cut

Rough alfredo sauce

1 cup cashews, sprinkled for in any occasion three hours (or medium-term) and exhausted 1/3 cup water

1 tsp agave or maple syrup

1 clove garlic

3-4 table spoon lemon juice (to taste)

1/4 cup dietary yeast

1/4 tsp sea salt

1. Utilize a spiralizer and cut the zucchini into various long strips.

2. Add the tomatoes and basil to the zucchini noodles and put them paying little mind to in a large mixing bowl.

3. Mix most of the alfredo sauce fixings in a fast processor till smooth.

4. Spread the paste in 1/2 cup sauce, and mix it in well, including additional sauce as required

Dull BEAN AND CORN BURGERS

Makes 4 Burgers

Fixings

1 tablespoon coconut oil

1 minimal yellow onion, divided

1 cup new, hardened or canned common corn bits

1 can regular, low sodium dull beans, drained (or 1/2 cups cooked dim beans)

1 cup dim shaded rice, cooked

1/4 cup oat flour (or ground, moved oats)

1/4 cup tomato stick

2 tsp cumin

One stacking tsp paprika

1 stacking tsp bean stew powder

1/2 - 1 tsp sea salt (to taste)

Dull pepper or red pepper, to taste

Method

1. Preheat your oven to 350 F.

2. Warmth the coconut oil in a large sauté compartment. Incorporate the onion and saute till onion is splendid, fragile, and fragrant (around 5-8 minutes).

2) Add corn, beans, and tomato paste to the compartment and warmth through.

3) Place the cooked rice into the bowl of a sustenance processor. Incorporate the beans, onion, tomato paste, and corn mix. Heartbeat to join. Incorporate flavors, oat flour, and a touch of water if you need it. Pulse more, until you have a thick and tenacious (yet flexible) mix. If the blend is exorbitantly wet, incorporate a tablespoon or two of additional oat flour.

4) Shape into 4 burgers and spot burgers on a foil-lined warming sheet. Warmth for 25 - 30 minutes, or until burgers are gently crisped, flipping once through. Present with new guacamole, at whatever point needed!

EGGPLANT ROLLATINI WITH CASHEW CHEESE

Serves 4

Fixings

For rollatini:

2 enormous eggplant, cut the long route into 1/4 inch thick cuts Olive oil

1/4 cups cashews, sprinkled for in any occasion three hours (or medium-term) and drained 1/2 tsp sea salt

1 little clove garlic, minced (optional)

2 table spoon lemon juice

1/3-1/2 cup water

1/4 cup dietary yeast

2 tsp dried basil

1 tsp dried oregano

Dull pepper to taste

1/2 10 oz. pack cemented spinach, defrosted and squashed by and large to empty all excess liquid (I press mine relentlessly through a strainer)

1/2 cups regular, low sodium marinara sauce

Procedure

1. Preheat barbecue to 400 F. Cut eggplants the long path into strips around 1/2" thick. Spot eggplant cuts onto getting ready sheets and sprinkle well with sea salt or fit salt. Let sit for

30 minutes; this decays sharpness and empties bounty soddenness. Pat the cuts dry, and shower them or brush them daintily with olive oil.

2. Broil eggplant cuts till singing (around 20 min), flipping almost through.

3. While eggplant is cooking, make the cashew cheddar. Detect the cashews, sea salt, garlic, lemon, and 1/3 cup water in a sustenance processor. Method till the mix is astoundingly smooth and fragile (you're going for a surface like creamy ricotta cheddar), stopping to scratch the bowl down a few times and including some extra water as fundamental. Stop the motor, and incorporate the new yeast, basil, oregano, and dim pepper. The system again to combine. Move the cashew cheddar to a bowl and mix in the cut spinach. Put the cheddar mix in a sheltered spot.

4. Expel the cooked eggplant from the barbecue and decrease warmth to 325 F. Empower the slices to cool until they can be dealt with. Move them to a cutting board and incorporate around 3 table spoon of the cheddar mix beyond what many would consider possible of one side. Climb from that side, and spot wrinkle down in a little supper dish. Repeat with every leftover cut.

5. Cover the eggplant moves with tomato sauce, and warmth, uncovered, for around 20-25 minutes, or until hot. Present with sides of the choice.

GINGER LIME CHICKPEA SWEET POTATO BURGERS

Makes 4-6 Burgers

Fixings

3/4 cup cooked chickpeas

1/2 little onion

1-inch ginger cut

1 tsp coconut oil

1/2 cups sweet potato, warmed or steamed and cubed 1/3 cup quinoa drops or sans gluten moved oats

Two heaping table spoon flax supper

2-3 table spoon lime juice (to taste)

2 table spoon low sodium tamari

1/4 cup cilantro, hacked

Run red pepper chips (optional)

Water as required

System

1. Preheat stove to 350 F.

2. Warmth coconut oil in a large dish or wok. Saute onion 2 tsp coconut oil (or coconut oil shower) till sensitive and fragrant (around 5 minutes). Incorporate chickpeas and warmth through.

3. Spot the chickpeas, ginger, and onion in a sustenance processor and incorporate the sweet potato, quinoa drops or oats, flaxseed, lime juice, cilantro, tamari or coconut aminos, and run of red pepper pieces, if using. Heartbeat to join, by then run the motor and incorporate some water until the consistency is thick yet direct to frame.

4. Shape mix into 4-6 burgers. Warmth at 350 degrees for around 35 minutes, flipping somewhat through.

SWEET POTATO AND BLACK BEAN CHILI

Serves 6

Fixings

1/2 cup dried dim beans.

5 cups sweet potato, diced into 3/4 inch shapes

One tablespoon olive oil

1/2 cups cut white or yellow onion

Two cloves garlic, minced

1 chipotle pepper in adobo, cut finely

2 teaspoons cumin powder

1/2 teaspoon smoked paprika

1 tablespoon ground bean stew powder

1 14 or 15-ounce container of typical, diced tomatoes (I like the Muir Glen brand)

1 can standard, low sodium dull beans (or 1/2 cups cooked dim beans)

2 cups low sodium vegetable soup, Sea salt to taste

Procedure

1. Warm the tablespoon of oil in a dutch stove or a huge pot. Saute the onion for at times, by then incorporate the sweet potato and garlic. Keep sauteing until the onions are sensitive, around 8-10 minutes.

2. Include the bean stew en adobo, the cumin, the stew powder, and the smoked paprika. Warmth until the flavors are extraordinarily fragrant. Incorporate the tomatoes, dull beans, and vegetable soup.

3. At the point when a stock is frothing, reduce to a stew and cook

4. Include progressively stock as required, and season to taste with salt. Serve.

1) Remaining bean stew can be set and will keep for up to five days.

CAULIFLOWER RICE WITH LEMON, MINT, AND PISTACHIOS

Serves 2

Fixings

5 cups unrefined cauliflower florets

1 oz pistachios

1/4 cup each basil and mint

2 tsp lemon flair

1/2 table spoon lemon juice

1 table spoon olive oil

1/4 cup dried currants

Sea salt and dim pepper to taste

System

1. Port 3 cups of the cauliflower to a sustenance processor. Methodology until the cauliflower is isolated into pieces that are about the size of rice. Move to a gigantic mixing bowl.

2. Move the remaining 2 cups of cauliflower to the sustenance processor. Incorporate the pistachios. The methodology, eventually until cauliflower is isolated into assessed rice pieces. Heartbeat in the basil and mint till herbs are finely hacked.

3. Include the extra separated cauliflower, pistachios, and herbs to the mixing bowl with the focal group of cauliflower. Incorporate the lemon squeeze, oil, and flows — season to taste with salt and pepper serve.

DULL COLOURED RICE AND LENTIL SALAD

Serves 4

Fixings

Two tablespoons olive oil

One tablespoon squeezed apple vinegar

One tablespoon lemon juice

1 tablespoon dijon mustard

1/2 tsp smoked paprika

Sea salt and dull pepper to taste

2 cups cooked dull hued rice

1 15-oz can typical, no sodium included lentils, flushed, or 1/cups cooked lentils

One carrot, diced or ground

4 table spoon severed fresh parsley

Strategy

1. Whisk oil, vinegar, mustard, paprika, lemon juice salt, and pepper together in a vast bowl.

2. Include the rice, lentils, carrot, and parsley. Mix well and serve

Rough "Shelled nut" NOODLES

Serves 2

Fixings

For the dressing:

One tablespoon ground ginger

1/2 cup olive oil

2 tsp sesame oil (toasted)

2 table spoon smooth white miso

Three dates, set, or ¼ cup maple syrup

1 table spoon Nama shoyu

1/4 cup water

For the noodles:

2 zucchinis

1 red ringer pepper, cut into matchsticks

1 carrot, ground

1 little cucumber, stripped into feeble strips

1 cup pitifully cut, steamed snow peas

1/4 cup cut scallions or green onion

System

1. Mix dressing fixings in a fast blender until all fixings are smooth and smooth.

2. Cut the zucchini into long, feeble "noodles." Combine the carrot with the pepper, zucchini, cucumber, and scallions.

3. Dress the noodles with enough dressing to cover them well. Serve.

Basic FRIED RICE AND VEGETABLES

Serves 2

Fixings

2 tsp toasted sesame oil

1 table spoon ground ginger

1/2 cups cooked darker rice

2-3 cups cemented or fresh vegetables of choice

1 table spoon low sodium tamari

1 table spoon rice vinegar

Vegetable squeezes as required

Procedure

1. Warmth the sesame oil in a large wok. Incorporate the ground ginger and heat it for a minute or two.

2. Include the dim shaded rice and vegetables. Saute till the vegetables are fragile.

3. Include the tamari, rice vinegar, and a sprinkle of vegetable stock if the mix is dry. Serve.

ARUGULA SALAD WITH GOJI BERRIES, ROASTED BUTTERNUT SQUASH, AND CAULIFLOWER

Serves 2

Fixings

For the plate of blended greens:

Fur stacking cups arugula (or other green)

1 lb butternut squash, stripped and separated

1 little head cauliflower, washed and separated into small florets

2 table spoon coconut or olive oil

Sea salt and pepper to taste

1/4 cup unrefined pumpkin seeds

1/4 cup goji berries

For the dressing:

3 table spoon olive oil

2 table spoon pressed the orange

1 table spoon lemon juice

1/2T tsp turmeric

1/4 tsp ground ginger

1 table spoon agave or maple syrup

Sea salt to taste.

Technique

1. Heave the cauliflower in the other tablespoon and season with salt and pepper. Cook the two veggies at 375 degrees for 20-

Thirty minutes (the cauliflower will cook faster), till splendid darker and fragrant. Oust from the stove and let it cool.

2. Spot the goji berries, arugula, and pumpkin seeds in a colossal bowl. Incorporate bubbled vegetables. Blend the olive oil, lemon juice, turmeric, maple syrup or agave, ginger together, and sea salt, and dress all of the veggies.

3. Gap serving of blended greens onto two plates, and serve.

COOKED VEGETABLE PESTO PASTA SALAD

Note: Instead of using dull hued rice or quinoa pasta in this dish, you can in like manner, mix the cooked vegetables and pesto into the whole grain, like darker rice or millet or quinoa, for a continuously healthy assortment.

Serves 4

Fixings

3 cups zucchini, severed into 3/4" pieces

3 cups eggplant, severed into 3/4" pieces

1 huge Jersey or fortune tomato, divided

2 tablespoon of olive oil or melted coconut oil

Sea salt and dim pepper to taste

8 oz dim shaded rice or quinoa pasta (penne and fusilli work honorably)

1/2 - 2/3 cup of walnut pesto

Procedure

1. Preheat your grill to 400F.

2. Lay the zucchini, eggplant, and tomato out on two material or foil fixed warming sheets and shower with the olive or coconut oil. Coat the vegetables with the oil and supper vegetables for thirty minutes or until sensitive and singing.

3. While vegetable cook, convey a pot of salted water to bubble. Incorporate the pasta and cook till still to some degree firm (according to package rules). Channel pasta and set aside in a deep mixing bowl.

1.   Add the cooked vegetables and to the pasta. Mix in the pesto, season to taste, and serve immediately.

PORTOBELLO "STEAK" AND CAULIFLOWER "Pureed potatoes."

Serves 4

Fixings

For the mushrooms:

1/4 cup olive oil

2 table spoon balsamic vinegar

2 table spoon low sodium tamari or nama shoyu

4 table spoon maple syrup

Sprinkle pepper

4 portobello mushroom tops, cleaned

Submerge 4 Portobello beat in the marinade. 1 hour will be adequate for them to be readied, yet medium-term in the fridge is incredibly better.

For the Cauliflower Mashed Potatoes:

1 cups cashews, rough

4 cups cauliflower, hacked into little florets and pieces

2 table spoon smooth white miso

3 table spoon healthful yeast

2 table spoon lemon juice

Sea salt and dull pepper to taste

1/3 cup (or less) water

Method

1. Spot cashews into the bowl of your sustenance processor, and technique into a fine powder.

2. Include the miso, lemon juice, dietary yeast, pepper, and cauliflower. Heartbeat to join. With the motor of the machine running, incorporate water in a pitiful stream, until the mix begins to take on a smooth, whipped surface. You may need to stop a significant part of an opportunity to clean the sides of the bowl and help it along.

3. At the point when the mix takes after pureed potatoes, stop, scoop, and serve close by a Portobello top.

QUINOA ENCHILADAS

Balanced from a recipe in Food52

Serves 6

Fixings

1 table spoon coconut oil

Two cloves garlic, minced

1 minimal yellow onion, severed

3/4 pounds kid Bella mushrooms, hacked

1/2 cup diced green bean stews

1/2 teaspoon ground cumin

¼ of teaspoon sea salt (or to taste)

One can common, low sodium dim beans or 1/2 cup cooked dim beans.

1/2 cup cooked quinoa

10 6-inch corn tortillas

1/4 cup common, low sodium tomato or enchilada sauce

Procedure

1. Preheat stove to 350 degrees.

2. In a colossal pot over medium warmth, warm coconut oil. Garlic and Sautee onion till onion is translucent (around 5-8 min). Incorporate mushrooms and cook until the liquid has been released and evaporated (another 5 min).

3. Add the bean stews to the pot and give them a blend for 2 minutes. Incorporate the cumin, sea salt, dull beans, and quinoa, and continue warming the mix until it's hot.

4. Lay a thin layer (1/2 cup) of marinara sauce in the base of a supper dish. Spot 33% of a cup of quinoa mix in the point of convergence of a corn tortilla and move it up. Detect the tortilla, wrinkle down, in the goulash dish. Repeat with each lingering tortilla, and after that, spread them with 3/4 cup of additional sauce. Get ready for 25 minutes and serve.

PASTERIES

BANANA SOFT SERVE

Makes 2 servings

Fixings

2 gigantic bananas, stripped and hacked into pieces, by then set 1/2 teaspoon vanilla

Technique

Spot bananas in a sustenance processor and turn the motor on. Allow the processor to continue running until the bananas have gotten continuously light, delicate, and smooth. They'll take after a smooth bowl of sensitive serve solidified yogurt!

You may need to stop two or multiple times to scratch the bowl down. Be patient and let the processor complete its duty — from the beginning, it'll show up as though the fragile serve isn't meeting up. However, it will. Present with any fixings you like: cacao nibs, diminish chocolate, nutty spread, divided nuts or seeds

Rough VEGAN BROWNIE BITES

Makes 24-30 balls

Fixings

2 cups walnuts

2/3 cup cacao nibs

Liberal crush sea salt (to taste)

1/4 cup rough cacao (or standard cocoa) powder

1/2 cups set dates

Methodology

1. Spot the walnuts, cacao nibs, sea salt, and cacao powder in a sustenance processor and method for certain occasions, or till everything is genuinely particularly squashed up.

2. Include the dates and methodology for an extra twenty seconds or close. The mix should remain together. If that it's not, keep taking care of until it remains together adequately when you press a little in your grip. If you need to, including several additional dates, will help integrate it.

3. Shape the "blend" into balls that are around 3/4 - 1 inch thick by moving it in your palms. Store in the icebox for 30 minutes, and from that point onward, they'll be set up to serve.

Unrefined, VEGAN VANILLA MACAROONS

Makes 15 macaroons

Fixings

1/2 cup unrefined almonds

One heaping cup unsweetened demolished coconut

1/4 cup coconut oil (will be most direct to climb the macaroons if the oil is healthy when you set it in the processor)

Three tablespoons maple syrup

1 teaspoon vanilla concentrate

Press sea salt

Technique

1. Add almonds to the sustenance processor and method till they're finely ground.

2. Include the remainder of the fixings and method again, till everything is particularly combined.

3. Working quickly (or else the coconut oil will mollify) crease the coconut mix into pretty much nothing (3/4" - 1") balls — spot on a material lined platter or warming sheet.

4. Move platter to the more relaxed, and refrigerate for a few hours, till the macaroons are solid. Serve.

Macaroons will keep in the fridge for whatever length of time that around fourteen days.

CHOCOMOLE

Serves 2

Fixings

1 immense, prepared Haas avocado, set

½ tsp vanilla

4 heaping tablespoons rough cacao powder

3 table spoon maple syrup or agave

1/4 cup water (more as required)

Methodology

Detect all fixings in a sustenance processor or Vitamix and blend till smooth. Serve.

BLUEBERRY GINGER ICE CREAM

Serves 2

Fixings

bananas

1 heaping cup set blueberries

1/2 inch new ginger (or 1/2 tsp ginger powder in the event that you're using a sustenance processor)

1/4 cup cashews

2 tsp lemon juice

2-4 table spoon almond or hemp milk

Technique

Blend all fixings in a quick blender. Start with 3 table spoon of almond milk and use the pack to endeavor to get the mix going without including an inordinate measure of liquid: you need a solidified yogurt, not a smoothie. If require an extra two tablespoons, use them, yet be patient and keep blending in with the pack till a thick consistency is practiced.

THE VEGAN MEAL RECIPES IDEAS

Vegetarian Meal Prep Recipes—Breakfasts, Lunches, Dinners, and Snacks!

We ought to be certifiable—eating great can be problematic. On the off chance that you fight to stay on track (as I do), dinner prep can be a help. Regardless, dinner prep can moreover feel like a lot of work… And, now and again comparative old plans get depleting. Unravel your prep and shake up you're everyday plan with these simple vegan dinner prep plans! (Additionally, most of them are in like manner VEGAN!)

Take a gander at these ten veggie-lover morning dinners, 10 snacks, 10 dinners, and 10 bites to see what you like. By then, you can mix and match to make TONS of new veggie lover supper prep blends! Collection in your dinner prep will keep sound sustenance charming! These plans are meatless, and the regular part is furthermore plant-put together for anyone conveying with respect to with a veggie lover lifestyle. Additionally, an enormous number of these veggie lover dinner prep plans are similarly sans gluten and without dairy!

Strong sustenance doesn't have to get debilitating. Besides, even minimal complex plans can be inconceivably tasty. A part of the veggie lover feast prep plans in this overview uses a couple of fixings! That is on the grounds that these plans are made with authentic, whole sustenances that outfit our bodies with the kind of fuel it increments in esteem. Moreover, it makes planning time a wreckless complex… Feel allowed to get innovative with different fixings and flavorings to make these veggie lover feast prep plans your own!

Kinds of Breakfast plans

#1: Freezer Oatmeal Cups

Not a medium-term oats fan? Feast prep your HOT cereal by partitioning and setting it into bread tins! Also, when you cook your group of grain, you can upgrade and improve it any way you like. In the mornings, warm two or three the cereal cups on the stove, or in the microwave. By then, mix in whichever new common item, nuts, or fixings that you like and appreciate! With such an enormous number of potential enhancements and mix-ins, you'll never have a debilitating breakfast!

#2: Pumpkin Spice Breakfast Cookies

Treats for breakfast?! Point of fact! These wonders are delightful sweet yet stacked with healthy fuel—with NO refined flours or included sugars! The pumpkin puree gives these treats a dash of normal sweetness. However, you are answerable for the sort and proportion of sugar you incorporate. In addition, using oats and oat flour keeps this supper prep breakfast whole grain and without gluten. Also, you can make this a veggie-lover breakfast by utilizing a flax egg and sans dairy chocolate chips or cacao nibs!

#3: Low Carb Crustless Quiche

Pie frame is tasty—no vulnerability about it. In any case, it's delivered utilizing refined flours that don't offer a ton of fuel for our bodies. Or maybe, you can set up your quiche straightforwardly into the pie dish! This recipe has a wool surface. However, it is up 'til now strong enough to cut into cuts.

Moreover, each cut has more than one serving of vegetables in it! Getting your veggies in has never been less complicated. It can now and again be difficult to find low carb veggie lover feast prep plans. In any case, this luscious quiche has only 5 grams of net carbs per serving!

#4: Superfood Smoothies

Concerning veggie lover feast prep plans, smoothies are a delightfully fundamental choice for a quick breakfast. Additionally, there are eternal flavor mixes you can examine! These five smoothie plans all contain too healthy foods that are stacked with cell fortifications and moderating benefits. Which superfood smoothie suits your style.

#5. Dangerous Cauliflower Brunch Bites

What do you gain when you cross a soft egg breakfast with another noon serving of blended greens? These scrumptious casual breakfast snack! Consolidate your fixings, incorporate your enhancements, and get ready in littler than anticipated scone tins. They're like infinitesimal covering fewer quiches! Moreover, you'd never deduce that one serving of these littler than regular bread rolls has an entire supper of CAULIFLOWER concealed inside! It incorporates some smoothness and thickness, notwithstanding immense measures of fiber and key nutrients!

#6: Mithai Overnight Oats

Here's a basic supper prep breakfast that recommends a flavor like a sweet DESSERT—a.k.a. "mithai" in Indian food! If you're burnt out on your equal old-same-old medium-term oats plan, this flavor combo is the perfect method to switch things up. They're sweet, rich, and stacked with moderate handling carbs to fuel you for the afternoon! Also, the pistachios and almonds incorporate some delightful protein and an incredible crunch. Make this your own with your most adored foods developed starting from the earliest stage. Or then again, combine some protein powder!

#7: Low Carb Pumpkin Bread

If you're scanning for in a rush veggie-lover dinner prep plans, this LOW-CARB pumpkin bread is the perfect other option! Stir up your player fixings, warmth, and you have a sound breakfast to last the entirety of your weeks. It's a direct supper that you can have arranged to get and go on involved mornings. Moreover, this fuel-filled breakfast uses no refined flours and is aggregate without sugar. Likewise, you can make this a Paleo breakfast by using a supported sugar.

#8: Quinoa Fruit Salad

Quinoa shouldn't be stunning ALL of the time—it adds sublime surface and sustenance to this sweet, essential breakfast! Quinoa is healthy, sans gluten grain that can augment an individual item serving of blended greens and keep you invigorated for the afternoon. Additionally, this superfood grain is in like manner high in protein and fiber! You can prepare an immense gathering of quinoa and hack your essential items close to the beginning of the week, one of the most direct veggie-lover supper prep plans on our overview.

#9: Three-Ingredient Pancakes

Now and again, the least unpredictable vegan dinner prep plans are the most superb. Additionally, you need 3 INGREDIENTS to make this healthy breakfast! These veggie-lover hotcakes are light, fluffy, and typically sweet with NO extra sugars—by the bananas. Prepare sure to use, spotted bananas for most extreme sweetness! Top with a liberal sprinkle of maple syrup and your favored fresh characteristic item.

#10: Mini Blueberry Blender Muffins

These little scale scones are SO typical to make—stir up your hitter, including blueberries, and warmth! Made with oats as opposed to refined flour, they're whole grain, fuel-filled, and without gluten. Additionally, the prepared bananas incorporate a trademark sweetness, so you might not need to include any sugar! It's grand in a rushed breakfast or a fundamental bite. In case you heat these into littler than typical scone tins, each shortbread is simply around 20 calories!

#11: Sweet Potato Coconut Curry Lentil Soup

Pick some plant-based protein into your lunch with this deliciously creamy soup. The coconut milk makes this soup satisfyingly thick and incorporates a segment of strong, fuel-filled fat. Likewise, it changes the kick of exuberant ginger and cayenne. Cooking vegetables in ghee makes them along for proficient heavenly flavor that you'll have to acknowledge over and over. However, you could use coconut oil or some other oil to make this a veggie-lover supper prep lunch!

#12: Curry Cauliflower Chickpea Bowl

Cauliflower is nutritious vegetables on earth, overflowing with fiber and infection, doing combating sulforaphane! Regardless, it can get a touch of depleting after quickly... Take your cauliflower to the following level with this appealing sweet curried dressing! Also, with the protein-squeezed chickpeas in this bowl, it's a significant feast prep lunch that will finish you off and keep you satisfied.

#13: BBQ Bean Salad

Dump the level plate of blended greens leaves and get-up-and-go things up with this BBQ bean serving of blended greens! The kidney beans are a mind-blowing wellspring of protein, fiber, and magnesium, which is a key mineral that can help deal with our rest cycle. Moreover, drenched in your most cherished BBQ sauce, it's a delicious sweet supper that never gets old. Also, canned beans and veggies keep this a SUPER diminished feast prep lunch! Try not to spare a moment to switch things up and use your favored vegetables.

#14: Chipotle Tofu Tacos

There are heaps of veggie lover dinner prep plans out there. However, what various will you endeavor? Make things less complicated on yourself with this ONE-PAN dinner! Covering your tofu in hummus and a short time later setting it up makes for a delightfully firm and energetic lunch. Moreover, joined with stewed veggies, it's a tolerable feast that is anything but difficult to prepare. Likewise, you can value the combo in any number of ways—stuffed into tacos, as a burrito bowl, or any way you like!

#15: Veggie-Packed Mac and Cheese Bites

Concerning mac and cheddar, by what method can you NOT go over the edge?! Luckily, you can warm your mac into little scale roll tins—the perfect kind of part control! The breadcrumbs make these wonders crisp ostensibly and deliciously soft inside. You can, in like manner, making this a sans gluten dinner prep lunch without gluten pasta and use oats as breadcrumbs. Best of all, each soft mac eat is packed with healthy veggies like cauliflower, carrots, and butternut squash!

#16: Sweet Potato Avocado and Black Bean Burrito

Skirt the standard slick burrito and endeavor this vegetarian burrito that is squeezed with healthy veggies! The sweet potato joins perfectly with the dull beans for a smooth, fiber-filled lunch. Besides, the avocado adds healthy monounsaturated fats to help keep you full! Every eats of this burrito is better than the last. Furthermore, you can make this a sans gluten lunch with a without gluten tortilla!

#17: Corn Chowder

This chowder is overflowing with yummy flavors like garlic, thyme, and paprika. Additionally, there's a hint of sweetness from the corn and coconut milk! In the blend, the coconut milk and potato make this chowder SO thick and satisfying. Additionally, you can cause a significant bundle to set, so you, for the most part, have a healthy dinner arranged!

#18: Meatless Bean "Meatballs"

Veggie lover meatballs?! Sounds like an amusing articulation, isn't that so? These meatless 'meatballs' make the unimaginable possible! Much equivalent to veritable meatballs, they're liberal, satisfying, and loaded down with protein. Regardless, that protein begins from nutritious BEANS as opposed to meat! Welcome them dunked in marinara, or over your favored pasta!

#19: Creamy Quesadilla

If you're looking for spending plan pleasant veggie lover feast prep plans, this quesadilla is a champ. One serving of this dinner costs under $1 to make! Squashed chickpeas and avocado make this vegan lunch effectively smooth. Furthermore, they add loads of fiber to keep you full for the afternoon!

Also, you can even sneak some nutrient-rich kale into your eating schedule. If you're not an enthusiast of kale, don't pressure—you won't taste it between all the smooth layers! Besides, instead of predominant reasoning, you CAN pack a quesadilla for lunch. It's brilliant warm or cold!

#20: BBQ Veggie Burger

Dim bean burgers can also be as healthy and finger-licking'- as extraordinary as any meat burger! Besides, these are so natural to make—make your blend, the structure into patties, and plan. These veggie burgers hold together genuinely well, so don't hesitate to pile them up with all the fix-ins. Regardless, as opposed to eggs, this equation uses oats as a spread, making these VEGAN veggie burgers! Likewise, you can prepare a group of patties and stop them for up to a quarter of a year. You can't beat 3-fixing vegan supper prep plans!

• CONCLUSION

Anyway, is intermittent fasting worth an attempt?

Definitely it is!

However, it most likely conflicts with all that you've been raised to accept.

Subsequently, "attempting it" won't feel like the proper activity.

However, in the wake of attempting it and encountering every one of the benefits, I promptly got dependent on it.

You may be pondering, "Great, if it's so useful for individuals, for what reason don't all the huge health and wellness businesses talk about it?"

… I'll reveal to you why…

Since intermittent fasting is FREE!

Except if something is gainful, the wellness business won't educate you regarding it.

How a lot of cash would the wellness business lose if individuals out of the blue started eating less?

Remember that the wellness business makes cash by selling you snacks, protein shakes, and a considerable amount of other stuff that you can use as one of your 6-8 little suppers.

This is the reason the 6-8 little dinners thing is so famous – It's PROFITABLE!

If everybody out of the blue started intermittent fasting, they wouldn't have to purchase "100 calorie snacks" to munch on for the day.

Consider it…

Instead, they'll pack their plates with all the more REAL food.

At the point when you have every one of those additional calories accessible for your dinners, you can eat twofold the servings of food and still lose weight.

Here and there throughout everyday life, you need to conflict with what you believe is correct and have a go at something different.

It's the best way to find new things that may be better for you.

Also, in case you're going to have a go at something new, I HIGHLY suggest beginning with this.

CPSIA information can be obtained
at www.ICGtesting.com
Printed in the USA
BVHW050731260421
605849BV00003B/349

9 781667 158532